BODY WEIGHT IN URBAN RICH ADULT WOMEN

By Anu T.

INDEX

ABSTRACT

The present cross-sectional observational study was carried out to determine factors associated with desirable body weight among adult urban affluent women in the reproductive age group. The study was conducted in two phases. During phase I (Quantitative data collection), urban affluent women (n=387) in the age group of 25-45 yrs with atleast one living child were studied for socio-demographic profile, health profile and co-morbidities, dietary history, dietary pattern, activity pattern, energy intake, energy expenditure and energy status. The subjects were assessed by questionnaire, anthropometric and body composition measurements. The 387 women were grouped into 4 BMI categories i.e N (normal; n=90), PO (at risk/pre-overweight; n=61), OW (over weight; n=156), and Ob (obese; n=80) on the basis of WHO (2004) classification for analysis of the factors affecting desirable body weight.

Socio demographic factors like younger age (p=0.001), less number of parity (p=0.001), nuclear family (p=0.002) were found to be significant for N.

Health profile factors like lower family history of NCD (p=0.001), normal weight status of parents (p<0.001), higher age of onset of menarche (p<0.001), higher age of marriage (p=0.001), higher age of parity (p<0.001), not using oral contraceptives (p=0.004), post-partum weight gain in the range of 3-4 Kg (p<0.001), self perceived normal weight status (p<0.001) and mean weight gain and loss in the range of 2-3 Kg per annum (p<0.001) were significant for N.

Significant dietary factors for N were ovo-vegetarian diet (p=0.001), regular consumption of three main meals in a day (p=0.001), fixed eating amount (p=0.001), eating preferably at fixed meal time (p<0.001), less frequency of eating out (p<0.001) and making smart food choices when eating out (p<0.001).

Factors related to physical activity found significant for N were lower mean sitting time ($p<0.001$), higher mean standing time ($p<0.001$), greater participation in household chores ($p<0.001$), greater indulgence in high energy expenditure activities while on holiday ($p=0.001$), preference for stairs even when there is a choice ($p<0.001$), lower mean sleeping time ($p=0.007$), lower television viewing time ($p<0.001$), more time spent with children ($p<0.001$), more time spent in exercise ($p=0.002$) and a PAL value of 1.69 ($p<0.001$). Also, out of the 24 women in the sample, who had a PAL value of > 1.75, 19 women (79.2%) were in N.

The multi-variate binary logistic regression analysis of these significant factors was carried out to identify the determining factors for desirable body weight. These determining factors were family history of obesity, hypertension and heart disease ($p<0.001$; OR=6.43), weight status of father ($p=0.006$; OR=3.44), self perceived normal weight status ($p<0.001$; OR=57.03), tendency to overeat when hungry ($p<0.001$; OR=17.55), longer sitting time ($p<0.001$; OR=2.5), and television viewing time ($p<0.001$; OR=1.013).

During phase II (Qualitative data collection), FGD was conducted to identify factors associated with desirable body weight, as well as those associated with weight gain/re-gain with the help of a set of 8-10 theme questions. Urban affluent women (25-45 yrs) participated in the FGD. A disciplined lifestyle, which included physical activity like pranayam/yoga along with fixed and regular eating pattern helped in maintaining normal weight. Whereas, longer sitting time, erratic and uncontrolled eating along with the role of the genes led to weight gain was expressed by the women in the study as **attributable** factors. FGD also revealed that certain weight management programs helped in reducing weight, but were unable to prevent weight re-gain, or were non sustainable.

Thus, the study helped in identifying dietary, behavioural and lifestyle factors important for maintaining desirable body weight among urban affluent women by both qualitative and quantitative approaches. The six significantly determining factors from quantitative study were in agreement from qualitative factors especially long sitting time, television viewing time and tendency to overeat as factors contributing to weight gain. The self perceived normal weight status (OR-57.03) brought significant behavioural changes, which were evident in FGD narrations also. It is quite possible that tracking one's own self image flags the sequel of behaviour changes which ensure normo weight status.

LIST OF ABBREVIATIONS

% TBW	percent total body water
AEE	activity energy expenditure
AHA	Americal Heart Association
ANOVA	analysis of variance
AT	activity thermogenesis
AUC	area under the curve
BEE	basal energy expenditure
BIA	bio-impedance analysis
BMI	body mass index
BMR	basal metabolic rate
CHD	coronary heart diseases
CHO	carboydérate
cm	centimeter
CVD	cardio-vascular diseases
d	day
DBP	diastolic blood pressure

LIST OF ABBREVIATIONS

DEXA	dual energy x-ray absorptiometry
dL	deciliter
DLW	doubly labelled water
EB	energy balance
EE	energy expenditure
EI	energy intake
En %	energy percent
FAO	Food And Agriculture Organization
FFM	fat free mass
FFMI	fat free mass index
FGD	focus group discussion
FM	fat mass
FMI	fat mass index
FPG	fasting plasma glucose
HC	hip circumference
HR	heart rate
HRM	heart rate method
hrs	hours
HSES	high socio economic status

LIST OF ABBREVIATIONS

Ht	height
ICMR	Indian Council of Medical Research
IOTF	International Obesity Task Force
Kcal	kilo calorie
Kg	kilogram
l	litre
LBM	lean body mass
LSES	low socio economic status
m	meter
min/d	minutes per day
MRI	magnetic resonance imaging
MSES	middle socio economic status
MUFA	mono unsaturated fatty acids
N	normal
n	sample size
NA	not applicable
NCD	non-communicable diseases
NCEP	National Cholesterol Eduction Programme
NEAT	non exercise activity thermogenesis

NFHS	National Family Health Survey
NFI	Nutrition Foundation of India
NHANES	National Health And Nutrition Examination Survey
NIN	National Institute of Nurition
NNMB	National Nutrition Monitoring Bureau
NS	non significant
Ob	obese
OR	odds ratio
OW	overweight
p	value of significance
PA	physical activity
PAL	physical activity level
PAR	physical activity ratio
PBF	percent body fat
PEM	protein energy malnutrition
PO	pre-overweight/at risk of overweight
PUFA	poly unsaturated fatty acids
r	Pearson's correlation coefficient
RDA	recommended dietary allowances

LIST OF ABBREVIATIONS

RMR	resting metabolic rate
ROC	Receiver Operating Characterictic curve
RWA	Residential Welfare Association
S	significant
SBP	systolic blood pressure
SD	standard deviation
T2DM	type 2 diabetes mellitus
TBW	total body water
TDEI	total day's energy intake
TEE	total energy expenditure
TEF	thermic effect of food
UNU	United Nations University
WC	waist circumference
WHO	World Health Organization
WHR	Waist to hip ratio
WSR	waist to stature ratio / waist circumference to height ratio
yrs	years

LIST OF TABLES AND FIGURES

LIST OF TABLES AND FIGURES

List of Figures

LIST OF ANNEXURE

CONTENTS

1. INTRODUCTION

The adult years are a broad span chronologically and, like all life cycle phases, are complicated by physiological, developmental and social factors. Along with their genetic and social history, adults have accumulated behavior and risks from environmental factors. These factors shape the heterogeneity of adult years. At the same time, adulthood is the ideal phase of the lifecycle for sensitivity to health promotion and disease prevention. Women have the potential to shape personal dietary and lifestyle choices and influence those of others. Nonetheless adult years are an ideal time for shaping a positive and a healthy old age.

In the transition from adolescence to early and then middle adulthood, health and wellness takes on a new importance. There is a sudden realization regarding one's own health. But this is also the time for the onset of various chronic degenerative diseases like CHD, hypertension, diabetes, etc. All these major chronic disease state have a direct relationship to unhealthy weight. Overweight and obesity in adults is a major risk factor in both the prevention and control of heart disease, stroke, diabetes, breast cancer, hypertension, etc.

Globally, 1.5 billion adults are overweight, of which over 200 million are men and nearly 300 million are women (WHO Facts Sheet, 2011). Data from India's Third National Family Health Survey (NFHS-3) conducted in 2005 – 2006 shows higher prevalence of overweight obesity in urban women vis a vis men. At the state level women of Punjab and Delhi rank first and second in the country's obesity count with 37% and 34% respectively, whereas the national average stands at 15% (NFHS-3, 2005-2006).

The concern for unhealthy weight is higher in women because apart from cosmetic disadvantage and obesity related co-morbidities, they are exposed to greater health risk like menstrual irregularities, pregnancy related complications, giving birth to overweight babies, ovarian cancer. Also women are more concerned about their weight status and are more likely to become overweight as they grow older (Sharan and Puttaraj, 2006).

In developing countries, obesity is concentrated in urban HSES women as compared to rural women due to high purchasing power, more accessibility to energy dense and fat rich foods and inactive life styles. This has resulted in calorie imbalance leading to weight gain. Indian women are not only gaining weight due to a shift in their life style but also they are born with adverse body composition features like at low BMI values they have high upper body adiposity and high body fat percentage (Kurpad, 2003). However, not all people exposed to this environment are obese. Therefore, other factors also have a role in development of obesity. Within this same socio-economic group and age group, there are women with healthy weight. Therefore, an insight onto the physical activity levels, dietary behavior and social life of women who have been able to maintain healthy weight versus those who have gained weight in the reproductive age group of 25-45 year will help to understand the role of various parameters on their body weight status.

Several studies in our lab have shown age related changes in energy expenditure, weight and body composition among women (Wasuja and Siddhu, 2002). Insight into body composition especially in Indian context is of paramount importance for monitoring weight maintenance among women (Sirohy et al, 2001; Siddhu, 2004)

Positive deviance factors in healthy eating practices, regular physical activity etc, which can contribute to maintenance of weight need to be studied and well established. This will help to formulate appropriate interventions by dietary and life style modifications.

This study delved deeper into overweight and obesity among urban affluent women. Co-morbidities were mapped. Diet and lifestyle of overweight and obese women were reviewed in relation to normal and pre-overweight women in the same community.

2. REVIEW OF LITERATURE

ETYMOLOGY (ORIGIN OF THE WORD)

The term obesity is derived from Latin word obesus, which in turn is a contraction of two Latin words, ob and edere, meaning to devour and to eat away. Its first attested usage in English was in 1651, in Noah Biggs's Matoeotechnia Medicine Praxeos (online etymology dictionary).

2.1 WHO INITIATIVE TO SOLVE THE OBESITY EPIDEMIC

The World Health Organization (WHO) International Obesity Task Force (IOTF) had defined obesity as a condition in which excess body fat adversely affects health and well being (WHO, 2000)[2].

The International Obesity Task Force (IOTF) was established in May, 1996 to tacle the emerging global epidemic of obesity.The IOTF initiative on the prevention and management of obesity has four main goals-

1. To increase the awareness among governments, health care professionals and the community that obesity is a serious medical condition and a major health problem with substantial economic costs.
2. To provide evidence and guidance for the development of both prevention and management strategies.
3. To secure the commitment of the policy makers to action.
4. To foster the development of international, national and regional structures that will enable and support the implementation of overweight and obesity.

WHO has developed the 2008-2013 Action plan for the global stratregy for the prevention and control of non-communicable diseases to help the millions, who are already affected, cope with these lifelong illnesses and prevent secondary complications. This action plan aims to build on the WHO Framework Convention ofn Tobacco Control and the WHO Global Stragegy on Diet, Physical Activity and

Health. The WHO Global Strategy on Diet, Physical Activity and Health describes the actions needed to support the healthy diets and regular physical activity. The Strategy calls upon all stake holders to take action at global, regional and local levels to improve diets and physical activity patterns at the population level. The action plant proves a road map to establish and strengthen initiatives for the surveillance, prevention and management of NCDs (WHO, 2011).

2.2 HISTORICAL TRENDS

The Greeks were the first to recognize obesity as a medical disorder (Haslam, 2007). Hippocrates stated that "corpulence is not only a disease itself, but the harbinger of others". It was known to the Indian surgeon Sushruta (6th century B.C.), who related obesity to diabetes and heart disorder. He recommended physical work to help cure it and its side effects. Foremost of human history, mankind struggled with food scarcity. With the onset of the industrial revolution, it was realized that the military and economic might of the nations were dependent on both the body size and strength of soldiers and workers. Increasing the average body mass index from underweight to the normal range played a significant role in the development of industrialized societies. Height and weight, thus both increased through the 19th century in the developed world. During the 20th century, as population reached their genetic potential for height, weight began to increase more than the height, resulting in obesity (Wikipedia encyclopedia).

2.3 WORLDWIDE TRENDS

The increasing trend of weight gain in the adult population has led to escalating obesity rates and to obesity being considered as one of the most serious public health challenges facing the world.

Obesity develops as a result of a complex interaction between a person's genes and the environment, characterized by long term energy imbalance due to excessive caloric consumption, insufficient energy output (sedentary lifestyle, low resting metabolic rate) or both (Afridi and Khan, 2004).

The WHO's projections indicate that approximately 1.6 billion adults (>15yrs) are overweight (BMI >25Kg/m^2) and at least 400million adults are obese (BMI >30Kg/m^2) globally. Also 20 million children under the age of 5years are overweight. The WHO projects that by 2015, approximately2.3 billion adults will be overweight and more than 700 million will be obese (WHO, 2005).

Secular trends show that the proportion of obese men increased from 3.4% in 1987 to 5.3% in 1992, while the proportion of obese women increased from 10.4% to 15.2% in the same period in Africa (WHO, 2000)[1]. Similarly, for USA, the NHANES III 1999, reported that the combined overweight and obesity prevalence in 20-74 year adults has risen from 50% to 61% since NHANES II 1988-1994 (WHO, 2003). Table 2.3.1 shows the prevalence of obesity for different regions of the world for both men and women.

Table 2.3.1 Obesity prevalence (BMI > 30) in different regions of the world and populations

Country or population	Year	Age (years)	Prevalence (%)	
			Men	Women
South Africa, (Blacks)	1990	15-64	8	44
USA	1988-1994	20-74	20	25
England (UK)	1995	16-64	15.0	16.5
Netherlands	1995	20-29	8.4	8.0
Malaysia	-	18-60	4.7	7.9
Japan	1993	20+	2.9	2.6
China	1992	20-45	1.2	1.6

- *Source: WHO (2000)*

Table 2.3.1 shows that the prevalence of obesity is Malaysia was 4.7% in men and 7.9% in women. WHO (2000)[1] reported that 17.1% women in India had a BMI over 30 as compared to 8.8% of Malay and 4.3% of Chinese women indicating that the problem of overweight and obesity is more serious in Indian population (WHO, 2000)[1].

Once considered a problem related to affluence, obesity is now fast growing in developing countries and countries in transition (WHO, 2000[2]; Shetty, 2001; WHO, 2003; Agrawal, 2005; Subramaniam and Smith, 2006; Roskam et al, 2010).

Even in countries like India, which are typically known for high prevalence of under nutrition, a significant proportion of overweight and obese people now coexist with those who are under nourished (Shukla et al, 2002; Popkin, 2002; Subramanian et al, 2009).

2.4 OBESITY IN INDIA

Obesity develops at any age, in either sex over time. However, in developing countries the overall incidence of obesity is higher among women than men (Mendez et al, 2005). In India, the problem of overweight/obesity is more profound among urban women (Gopalan, 1989; Wasuja and Siddhu, 2002; Venkatramna, 2002; Agrawal and Mishra, 2004; Aggrawal, 2005; Bhadra, 2005; Garg et al, 2010).

Currently, India is in nutrition transition with 10% rural adults and 20% urban adults suffering from over-nutrition and an emerging double burden of malnutrition (Gopalan, 2008). The National Family Health Survey (NFHS-3, 2005-2006) reported that 15% of ever married women are overweight or obese, which is up from 11% which was reported in NFHS-2, 1998-1999. It was also reported, based on all India data, that the problem of over nutrition was higher among women with a prevalence of 15% as compared to 12% in men.

The problem of overweight / obesity was more among urban women , well educated women and women belonging to HSES. Sikh women showed higher prevalence of obesity (NHFS-3, 2005-2006; Garg etal, 2010). At the state level urban women of Punjab and Delhi rank first and second in the country's obesity count with 37.5% and 34% respectively. Table 2.4.1 depicts the prevalence of obesity in India and in Delhi, in ever married adults (15-49 years) according to NFHS-III (2005-2006).

Table 2.4.1 NFHS- III Data on prevalence of obesity in adults (2005 – 2006)

Category	NFHS-III (All India)	Residence		NFHS-III (Delhi)
		Urban	Rural	
Women who are overweight or obese (BMI ≥ 25)	14.8%	28.9%	8.6%	32.9%
Men who are overweight or obese (BMI ≥ 25)	12.1%	22.2%	7.3%	24.0%

The table 2.4.1 shows that more women are obese as compared to men, irrespective of their residence in urban or rural areas. In Delhi, about 33% of women are obese as compared to 24% of men.

An epidemiological study of obesity in adults in urban population of Delhi reported an overall prevalence rate of obesity as 27.8%. Obesity was found to be 21.3% among males and 33.4% among females; $p<0.001$ (Gopinath et al, 1994).

Gopalan (1998) reported the following obesity prevalence: upper strata 32.0% (male) and 50.0% (female), middle class 16.2% (male) 30.3% (female), LSES 7.0% (male) and 27.8% (female), poor urban slum 1.0% (male) 4.0% (female).

In another study by Reddy et al (2002), it was reported that 35% of adult males and 48% of adult females are obese in urban Delhi.

Shukla et al (2002) reported that 19% of males and 30% of females were obese in Mumbai.

Zargar et al (2000) reported an obesity prevalence of 23.7% in females and 7.0% among males in the Kashmir Valley.

Varghese and Vijayakumar (2008) reported that 30-40% of the subjects in the most productive age group (30-50years) were either obese or overweight in a rural setting in Kerala.

Bhadra et al (2005) reported 37.34% overweight (BMI 25-30) and 17.45% obese (BMI>30) among Hindu, Bengalee women of Kolkata.

2.5 OBESITY AND HEALTH

Regardless of its cause, obesity may be associated with a variety of risks. Obesity causes or exacerbates many health problems, both independently and in association with other diseases (WHO, 2003).

Epidemiological evidence also links obesity to increased morbidity and mortality and increased risk of chronic diseases. In 2001, globally non-communicable conditions, including CHD, diabetes, obesity, cancers, and respiratory diseases, accounted for 59% of the 56.5 million deaths and 45.0% of the global burden of disease. The proportion of burden is expected to increase to 57% by 2020 (WHO, 2003). Of 17 million deaths, the majority were related to heart disease and stroke. This reflects a shift in the pattern of disease worldwide, so many countries in the developing world are now struggling with the double burden of both infectious and non-communicable diseases. This shift in turn reflects a significant change in dietary habits, physical activity levels, and tobacco use as a result of industrialization, urbanization, economics development, and the increasing globalization of food market (Waxman, 2003). It has been projected that the number of people in the developing world with diabetes will increase from 84 million in 1995 to 228 million in 2025. On a global basis, 60% of the burden of chronic disease will occur in developing countries (WHO, 2003).

Obesity is a first step, a gateway, to the chronic diseases. Hypertension, Hypercholesterolemia, Heart Disease, T2DM, Gall Bladder Disease, Asthma, Mental Health concerns – Depression, Low Self Esteem and Orthopedic Disorders, have all been linked to obesity (Agrawal and Mishra, 2004; American Academy of Pediatrics, 2003; WHO, 2003).

2.5.1 Obesity and CHD

CHD is an important cause of morbidity and mortality in most industrialized nations, and is gaining importance as a major disease in developing countries as well. The emerging evidence of the CHD epidemic in developing countries, including India, is significant to suggest that people of South Asian origin are more prone to CHD. About 40 million people in India suffer from CHD (Gupta et al, 2003) with a prevalence of 7-10% in North Indian urban adults and 14% in urban South Indian adults (Mohan et al, 2001). One of the cardinal features of CHD prevalence is the marked prematurity resulting in a greater risk at younger ages supported by the data that in comparison to whites, the relative risk of CHD mortality is 1.77 times higher in Indians between the ages of 20-29 years (Reddy and Yusuf, 1998; Reddy et al, 2002). Mc-Tigue et al (2003) reported that weight gain of 5-8 Kg increased CHD risk by 25% and weight gain of 20 Kg increased the risk more than 2.5 times compared to women whose weight was stable within 5 Kg range.

Dyslipidemia is also associated with obesity. The LDL-cholesterol levels increase by 10-20 mg/dl with increase in BMI from 20 to 30 Kg/m^2 (Jain, 2005).

2.5.2 Obesity and hypertension

Hypertension is very common in individuals who are obese. It is generally believed that people who are overweight are 2 to 3 times more likely to have elevated blood pressures. According to the results of a meta-analysis, a weight loss of 1.0 Kg is associated with a decrease of 1.2 – 1.6 mm Hg in systolic blood pressure and 1.0 – 1.3 mm Hg in diastolic blood pressure (WHO, 1995). Body fat thus seems to be linearly related to increase in blood pressure and prevalence of hypertension. It has been estimated that a 5% decrease in blood pressure can reduce the rate of stroke by 34% and that of CHD by 21% (Rao and White, 1993).

Gupta (2004) reported a prevalence of hypertension in 27% male and 28% female executives in Mumbai, whereas in Jaipur it was reported as 36% for men and 37% for women. Hypertension prevalence was found to be lower in rural Indian population, although there has been a steady increase over time. Yajnik (2002) explained that changing lifestyle factors are responsible for the occurrence of cardiovascular diseases in the Indian community.

Mertens and Gaal (2008) reported weight gain in adult life as an important risk factor for the development of hypertension. The co-relation of hypertension with obesity is most marked in young men and women with abdominal obesity (Jain, 2005).

2.5.3 Obesity and diabetes

Obesity has long been known to be associated with type-2 diabetes mellitus (T2DM). The risk of type-2 diabetes mellitus (T2DM) increases as BMI increases (Gastaldelli, 2008). Approximately 80% of patients with this form of disease are obese (WHO 1995). The evidence for this comes from the data showing that the prevalence of diabetes in the US has increased to exactly the same extent as that of obesity, from 5.76 per million in 1980 to 12.0 per million in 2000 (Marsh, 2003). The prevalence of diabetes ranges from 2% in rural Indian communities to 1% in urban Indian cities and upto 16% in migrant Indians (Simmons et al, 1992). According to the Diabetes Atlas, 2006 published by the International Diabetes Federation, the number of people with diabetes in India currently around 40.9 million is expected to rise to 69.9 million by 2025 (Mohan et al, 2007). The occurrence of diabetes within a community appears to be triggered by a number of environmental factors such as sedentary lifestyle, dietary factors, stress, urbanization and socio economic factors. The summary of the WHO World Health Report (2002) estimates that two-thirds of the estimated 177 million people worldwide affected by diabetes (mostly type 2) live in the developing world (Waxman, 2003).

2.5.4 Obesity and metabolic syndrome

Persistent obesity dysregulates metabolic processes including action of insulin on glucose-lipid-free fatty acid metabolism and severely affects processes controlling blood glucose, blood pressure and lipids. Thus, begins a cluster of conditions; dysglycemia, dyslipidemia, hypertension and procoagulant state, known as the metabolic syndrome (Grundy, 2003). Data suggests that obesity and metabolic syndrome are immediate precursors of type-2 diabetes mellitus and cardio-vascular disease (NCEP, 2002; Mensah et al, 2004).

In line with the rising prevalence of obesity, the metabolic syndrome is also increasing in developing countries (Popkin, 2006). High prevalence of the metabolic syndrome has been reported from Sub-Saharan Africa and Middle East countries; South Africa, Morocco, Oman, Turkey and Iran showed prevalence of 33.5, 16.3, 21, 33.4 and 33.7 per cent respectively (Lafta and Kadhim, 2005; Kruger et al, 2006; Silveira et al, 2006).

The situation is quite similar in South Asian countries. The data shows that one fourth to one third of urban population of India has the metabolic syndrome (Misra and Khurana, 2008). The prevalence is 1.5 to two time higher in women compared with men. Also, certain communities in India like Punjabi Bhatia Community in North India have inordinately high tendency to have obesity, type-2 diabetes mellitus and metabolic syndrome (Gupta et al, 2004).

2.5.5 Obesity and women's health

Obesity or significant overweight can contribute many problems in women's reproductive system, like prolonged or heavy periods, menstrual pains, delayed ovulation, mid cycle spotting, short luteal phase, pre-menstrual spotting, pre-menstrual syndrome (PMS), infertility, amenorrhea, fibroids, tumor of uterus, breast cancer, endometrial cancer, ovarian cancer, uterine prolapse (Agrawal, 2005).

In a cross-sectional population based study on 2225 subjects aged ≥ 20 yrs in Chandigarh city in North India on prevalence and risk factors of metabolic syndrome among Asian Indian by Ravikiran et al (2010) revealed that the risk factors for metabolic syndrome are increasing age, sedentary lifestyle, female gender and diabetes in parents. Thus highlighting that occurance of metabolic syndrome which is closely linked to obesity is higher among women. It has been estimated that upto 80% of cases of CHD, 90% of type 2 diabetes and one third of cancers of all types can be avoided by changing to a healthier diet, increasing physical activity, and decreasing tobacco consumption (Waxman, 2003).

Weight loss can reverse or arrest the harmful effects of obesity. Lifestyle intervention studies have shown the effectiveness of weight loss in improving cardiovascular risk factors, including blood pressure, insulin resistance, type-2 diabetes, lipid disorders and metabolic syndrome in population at high risk for such diagnoses (Klein et al, 2004).

2.6 OBESITY AND SOCIO-ECONOMIC STATUS (SES)

Patterns of prevalence of overweight and obesity have emerged across different socio-economic groups. In developed countries levels of obesity are higher in the lower socio-economic groups. In developing countries this relationship is reversed. Several researchers in their studies have reported that for both men and women there is an increasing proportion of a positive association and a decreasing proportion of negative association as one moved from countries with high levels of socio-economic developments to countries with medium and low levels of development (Sobal and Stunkard, 1989; Shukla, 2002; WHO, 2003; Mc Laren, 2007; Dahly et al, 2010). Subramanian et al (2009) observed a positive relationship between socio-economic status and BMI, in India.

In a cross-sectional analysis of nationally representative samples of 538140 women aged 15-49 years drawn from 54 Demorgaphic and Health surveys conducted between 1994 and 2008, it was observed that globally, a one-quartile increase in wealth was associated with a 0.54 increase in BMI (95% CI: 0.50, 0.64) and 33% increase in overweight (95% CI: 26%, 41%) in adjusted models. The association between wealth and BMI and overweight was positive in 96% (52 of 54) of the countries (Subramamian et al, 2011)

India is in a unique position of its epidemiological and nutritional transition due to its huge population and extremes of economic conditions. The factors contributing to rising obesity rates include large scale societal and nutritional changes due to modernization and globalization of food markets (WHO, 2003; Hawkes, 2005; Hawkes, 2006; Mc Laren, 2007).

Transition is evident in the high socio-economic society in India to westernized lifestyle, which is incompatible with their evolutionary development. Also, sudden economic growth and globalization has led to increased availability of fat rich energy dense foods (Misra etal, 2005).

2.7 OBESITY, GENDER AND AGE

Clear gender differences are seen in most countries with more women than men being obese (Zargar at al, 2000; James et al, 2000; Filizof et al, 2001; Mokhtar et al, 2001; Ismail etal, 2002; Mc. Laren, 2007). WHO in its updated facts sheet on obesity and overweight in March 2011 reported that out of 1.5 billion overweight adults, 200 million men and 300 million women were obese (WHO, 2011). Research on obesity in India has found prevalence to be higher among HSES women (Shukla et al, 2002; Agrawal and Mishra, 2004; Bhadra, 2005; Sinha & Kapoor, 2009). Various cross sectional studies have reported weight gain especially in women in the 30-40 years age group and that the BMI of women increases with parity (Nagpal and Siddhu, 1996; Sirohy et al, 2001; Wasuja and Siddhu, 2002).

Data from India's Third National Family Health Survey (NHFS-3) conduced in 2005-2006 shows higher prevalence of overweight/obesity in women vis a vis men.

Del et al (2002) explained that the gender difference in the prevalence of obesity is due to the difference in the brains response to hunger and satiety in men and women.

In a study of obesity among North Indian women it was found that women working as professional technical/managers were prone to be overweight and obese than those working in other fields (Agrawal, 2002; Agrawal, 2005).

Age wise, a significant increase has also been noticed for obesity. In developed countries it has been found that there occurs an increase in body weight with ageing, atleast upto 50-60 years old. The relationship between obesity and age is similar in developing countries, but the maximum rate of obesity tend to be reached at an earlier age, i.e. upto 40 years (Agrawal, 2002; Shukla, 2002; Wasuja and Siddhu, 2002; Agrawal, 2005). This increase in age related weight and body fat in women can be modulated by exercise among normo-weight women (Sirohy et al, 2001).

2.8 OBESITY AND URBANISATION

Urban residence significantly increases the risk of obesity as reported in various research studies (Shukla et al, 2002; Yajnik, 2004; Agrawal & Mishra, 2004; Mendez etal, 2005; Bhadra, 2005; Agrawal, 2005). The transition from a rural to an urban lifestyle is associated with increased levels of obesity, which has been linked with dramatic changes in lifestyle, i.e. increased consumption of high energy dense foods and decrease in physical activity (Gopalan, 1998).

Urban rural differences in the prevalence of obesity are also evident in the study by NFI in which it was reported that prevalence rate of obesity was 32.2% and 50% in HIG males and females respectively, as compared to 1% and 4% for male and female urban slum dwellers respectively (Gopalan, 1998).

Subramanian et al (2011) observed a positive association between urbanization and overweight status in a cross-sectional analysis of 54 Demographic and Health Surveys conducted between 1994 to 2008.

Urban residence and higher income were associated with lower energy intake, higher fat intake and lower physical activity level compared to rural residence and other income categories (WHO, 2003; Mc. Laren, 2007). Urbanization involves changes in dietary pattern, occupation patterns, lifestyle, and family structures. These changes have an impact on dietary intake and levels of physical activity.

2.9 ETIOLOGY OF OBESITY

The etiology of obesity is complex and multi-factorial. Obesity arises as a consequence of how the body regulates energy intake, energy expenditure and energy storage. The imbalance between food intake and energy expenditure can be due to biological, behavioral and environmental factors.

(I) Biological factors include genetics and biological response to energy intake.

(a) Genetics – Predisposition to obesity is inherited as reported from study of twins (Prentice, 2005). Many of the hormonal and neural factors involved in weight regulation are determined genetically. These include the short and long term signals that determine satiety and feeding activity. Small defect in their expression or interaction contribute significantly to weight gain (Frayling et al, 2007). The number and size of fat cells, regional distribution of body fat and RMR are influenced by genes (Gee et al, 2008). Although, the contribution of genetic factors to obesity is not clear at the population level, however a number of rare syndrome of extreme obesity have been related to specific mutations in genes (Barsh et al, 2000).

(b) Biological response/Metabolic susceptibility – All mature animals including humans, have biological systems that help match energy intake with energy expenditure to achieve energy balance to stabilize body weight. The human body is biologically geared to protect itself more strongly against weight loss than against weight gain. This biological defense is higher in certain group of people as compared to others (Hill, 2006).

(II) Behavioural factors – The rise in obesity level cannot solely be attributable to our biology. Changes in our diet and physical activity can lead to weight gain.

(a) Diet – Dietary composition, which includes more saturated fat and less fiber is accodicated with obesity (WHO, 2003). Urban diets includes superior grains, more milled and polished grains, higher fat content, more animal products, more sugar and more prepared and processed food (Prentice, 2001). In a study on 629 Indian females in the age group of 13-25 years, for their dietary profile and anthropometry by

Gupta et al (2010), revealed that the total fat intake was four times the recommended allowance. Also, there was an increased intake of milk, milk produces, roots and tubers. The study also reported that out of the total fat intake, the intake of saturated fat was higher than MUFA and Omega – 3 PUFA. These imbalances in the dietary intake might be responsible for the increasing prevalence of obesity.

(b) Physical activity – The effect of eating more calories is compared by low energy expenditure leading to positive energy balance and thus weight gain. Now a days, people are exercise less and spending more time in low energy activities such as watching television, using computer and driving to work place (WHO, 2003; Levine et al, 2006). This has contributed largely to the global obesity epidemic..

(III) Environmental factors – Although obesity has a genetic etiology, the major precipitating factor is environment, mostly related to sedentary lifestyle, which leads to conservation of energy as body fat (Snehlatha et al, 2003). Our external environment has great power in promoting obesity. Both the food and physical activity environment have changed over times in a way to encourage over eating and discourage physical activity (Hill and Peters, 1998; Hill et al, 2003).

(a) Food environment – In the present scenario food is high in fat and sugar. It is inexpensive and available in large portions. Food is heavily advertised and has become acceptable to have food everywhere (Hill, 2006).

(b) Physical activity environment / Built environment – Our physical activity environment has changed largely due to technological advances that make it unnecessary to be physically active in our daily lives. Most occupations no longer involve physical activity, and we no longer need to be physically active for transportation. The development of television, computers, the internet and video games has filled our leisure time with sedentary rather than physically active pursuits. These days, town planning promotes driving and not walking (AHA, 2008). Urban planning necessitates long commutes and restricts opportunities for walking. Also, there is limited and/or unsafe public spaces for recreational acticvity and pervasive presence of food outlets and opportunities to eat, usually fast, energy dense foods has led to increased obesity prevalence (Frank et al, 2004).

2.10 MEASURES OF OBESITY

2.10.1 Body weight and body composition

Bodyweight is the sum of bone, muscles, organs, body fluids and adipose tissue (Karelis et al, 2004). Therefore, body composition can be best understood in terms of four compartment model.

Body components can be broadly divided into two groups – fat mass (FM) and fat free mass (FFM) (Wagner and Heyward, 2000). During obesity, the fat mass increases inn greater proportion than fat free mass be it lean body mass, water or bones.

2.10.2 Body mass index and body weight

A WHO sponsored expert consultation on obesity advocated the use of BMI to determine the weight status of individuals (WHO, 2000[1]; WHO, 2004). It was suggested that this would permit meaningful comparison of weight status within and between populations, the identification of individuals and group at increased risks of morbidity and mortality, identification of priority for intervention at the individual or the community level and a firm basis for evaluating interventions (WHO, 2000[1]).

Studies have shown that BMI is a reasonable index of adiposity because body weight and stature are simple, inexpensive, safe and practical measurements to acquire, particularly for groups with limited access to health care (Gallagher et al, 1996; Fernandez et al, 2003; Daniels, 2009).

It can be used by the general public to assess a person's risk for chronic diseases and illness because BMI is easily calculated and therefore accessible to the lay person (Seidell et al, 2001).

Overweight and obesity are commonly defined by the measurement of BMI. Results of several studies have shown that BMI correlates highly with percentage body fat and is largely independent of height enabling an unbiased comparison between short and tall population groups (Norgan, 1994; Gallagher et al, 1996).

2.10.3 BMI cut-off values for Asian Indians

The umbrella term Asian characterizes a vast and diverse portion of the world's population. Diversity in Asian countries is based on ethnic and cultural sub groups, degrees of urbanization, social and economical conditions and nutritional transition. Asian population covers a wide range of morbidity and mortality profile, social and economic determinants of health (WHO, 2004). Various research studies have reported that Asians have lower mean BMI with high body weight percentage than non Asian population (Kurpad, 2004; Siddhu, 2004; WHO, 2004; Rush et al, 2009; Taylor and Goto, 2007; Misra et al, 2009). At the international level WHO (1995) recommended BMI cut-off points are used for comparisons across the globe. But from the Asian population perspective, the validity and relevance of these cut-off points has been questioned by various researchers (Ko et al, 2001; Misra, 2003; Siddhu, 2004; Singh et al, 2008). The WHO (2004) expert consultation concluded that the proportion of Asian people with a high risk of type-2 diabetes and cardio-vascular disease is substantial at BMIs lower than the existing WHO cut-off points for overweight i.e 25 Kg/m^2. The cut-off point for observed risk varies from 22 Kg/m^2 to 25 Kg/m^2 in different Asian populations and for high risk it varies from 26 Kg/m^2 to 31 Kg/m^2. The consultation, however, recommended that the current WHO (2004) BMI cut-off points should be retained as the international classification, but realized the significance of lowered cut-off points for obesity in the Asia Pacific region. The WHO (2004) consultation also recommended the cut-off points of 23, 27.5, 32.5 and 37.5 Kg/m^2 as points for public health action.

2.10.4 Percent body fat (PBF)

Since obesity is defined as excess accumulation of fat in the adipose tissue, therefore it becomes imperative to study the percent body fat for the purpose of risk stratification (Singh et al, 2008). The measurement of body fat that is composed of adipose tissue in the form of triglycerides represents a challenge to researchers and clinicians. The main stores of fat are subcutaneous and intra-abdominal, and an accumulation of an excess of body fat may adversely affect the health (Willet et al, 1999). A more accurate definition of overweight and obesity should be more appropriately based on the total amount of body fat due to the ethnic differences in height, weight, architecture and proportion of bones, muscles and fat (Dudeja et al, 2001; Piers et al, 2003). The incidents of impaired insulin sensitivity was reported to be 40% among women with PBF>30 but with normal BMI (Dvorak et al, 1999). The risk of co-morbidities is reported to be higher among South Asians (Indians, Pakistanis and Bangladeshi) at a lower BMI range than Caucasians (Shetty, 2002). In another study, 66% non-obese Asian Indian men were found to be insulin resistant due to a high body fat and low muscle mass (Banerji et al, 1999). Hence, it was shown that BMI has poor sensitivity and positive predictive value in identifying overweight/obese individuals when classified by body fat percentage (Siddhu, 2004)

2.10.5 Role of ethnicity and PBF

Ethnic differences in the relation between BMI and PBF have now been well reported. More specifically, at the same BMI, PBF differed between Asian, African-American and white person after age, sex, height and weight were controlled (Deurenberg-Yap et al, 1998; Gallagher et al, 2000)

Asian Indians have a characteristic obesity phenotype, consisting of –

- Shorter height and lower BMI as compared with whites or blacks;
- Higher body fat per unit BMI;

- Abdominal adiposity indicated by high WHR, normal waist circumference as compared with whites or blacks and high intra abdominal fat;

- Truncal adiposity is high as indicated by the sub-scapular skin fold thickness and more abdominal subcutaneous fat as compared with whites or blacks.

(Yagnik, 2004; Siddhu, 2004; Misra and Vikram 2004; Mohan et al, 2007).

Excess body fat and lesser amount of lean tissue compliments each other in volume and weight so that the value of BMI does not increase (Yagnik, 2004; Bisla et al, 2009). So, BMI alone does not indicate the true weight status for Asian Indians because it is calculated by combined estimates of fat, bone, muscles and body water (Dudeja et al, 2001; Piers et al, 2003). Therefore, variations in any of these components due to pathological or physiological perturbations would alter the value of BMI. In Asian Indians, the relative contribution of fat is more and muscle is less, therefore in such a situation, obesity should be studied with respect to body fat.

The body fat contents varies with socio economic status, dietary habits, activity profile, age, height, weight and ethnicity (Misra et al, 2003; Siddhu, 2004; Singh et al, 2008; Rust et al, 2009). Some other workers have also observed a high PBF in Asian Indians at a comparatively low BMI. In a study carried out on migrant Indian male volunteers in USA, the mean BMI of 25.0% Kg/m^2 was associated with 33% PBF (Banerji et al, 1999). Similarly, in urban Asian Indian females the prevalence of overweight according to PBF estimation was more than twice that estimated by BMI (Dudeja et al, 2001). The relationship between the amount of body fat and BMI is steeper in Asians, particularly Indians (Dudeja et al, 2001; Yap et al, 2002).

The cut-offs for body fat for different ethnic groups have not yet been validated and different authors have categorized individuals based on separate criteria as revealed from Table 2.10.5.

Table 2.10.5 Suggested PBF levels at varying BMI							
Reference	**Women PBF (%)**			**Men PBF (%)**			**Ethnicity**
	BMI ≤ 18.5	**BMI 25-30**	**BMI > 30**	**BMI ≤ 18.5**	**BMI 25-30**	**BMI > 30**	
Gallagher et al, 2000	21	33	39	8	21	26	Whites (20-39 y)
Deurenberg et al, 1991	-	-	30	-	-	25	Caucasians
Lean et al, 1995	-	34	-	-	22	-	Scottish
Zhu et al, 2003	22.5	30.8	37.2	11.0	21.2	29.1	White
Zhu et al, 2003	25.4	32.0	37.1	12.7	21.7	28.3	Black
Gallagher et al, 2000	25	35	40	13	20	26	Asian (20-39 y)
Gallagher et al, 2000	20	32	38	8	20	26	African-American (20-39 y)
Siddhu, 2004	-	35	-	-	-	-	Young Indian Females (MSES)
Kurpad, 2005	-	29	36	-	24	32	Indian LSES

The limits of body fat for defining obesity, although still debatable, have been set by different researchers for different ethnic groups. Empirically identified limits, population percentile, and z-scores have all been suggested as means of setting body fat percent guidelines, although each has major limitation (Gallagher et al, 2000).

2.10.6 Abdominal obesity/Central obesity

Various epidemiological studies have reported that it is important to study the location or distribution of fat in the body to understand the relation of obesity to various metabolic disturbances (Wachenberg, 2000; Kurpad, 2005). The criterion for clinical diagnosis of abdominal obesity has been the use of waist hip ratio (WHR). A WHR of > 1.0 for men and > 0.85 for women has been accepted as an indicator of abdominal obesity (Shetty, 2000). However, abdominal fat mass in any individual can vary for the same BMI and for the same amount of total body fat. This is evident from the results of NFI study, showing that 19% of non-overweight males (BMI < 25) have abdominal obesity (Gopalan, 1998).

Various research studies have reported that excess fat in the central (visceral abdominal) versus peripheral part of the body (Gluteofemoral) is associated with higher plasma glucose and insulin, hyperlipidemia and decreased HDL cholesterol concentration, components of insulin resistance syndrome and constituting a cluster of risk factors for atherosclerotic cardiovascular disease (Wachenberg, 2000; Garg, 2004; Karla et al, 2009; Zaher et al, 2009). Therefore, abdominal obesity is considered to be a more reliable indicator of metabolic syndrome than BMI. Evidence from a study by Zhu et al (2003) using the Third National Health and Nutrition Examination Survey Data in 9019 whites reported that waist circumference (WC) is more closely linked to cardio-vascular disease risk factors than is BMI. Similarly, Vikram et al (2003) reported a high prevalence of abdominal obesity in the Indian urban slum dwellers by WHR criterion as compared to 3-8% by WC cut-off values as defined by WHO (1995).

Waist circumference is an aggregate measurement of total and abdominal fat accumulation and is a crucial correlate of homeostatic mechanisms found among overweight patient (Wang, 2003). Therefore, measurement of WC provides a simple and practical method of identifying overweight patients at an increased risk of obesity related metabolic disorders. WC>102 cm for men and WC>88 cm for women have been recommended by NIH expert panel for identifying the increased relative risk for obesity co-morbidities for most adults with BMI > 25 Kg/m^2 (Han et al, 1995; Lean et al, 1995; NIH, 1998).

The results of the study of a Dutch population by Han et al (1995) suggests that action levels based on waist measurements may provide a valuable and simple method for alerting people at increased risk of cardiovascular disease. They suggested that WC exceeding 94 cm in men and 80 cm in women correctly identified subjects with BMI $\geq$ 25 and WHR $\geq$ 0.95 in men and $\geq$ 0.080 in women with a sensitivity and specificity of ≥ 96%. This study is supported by the findings of various other research studies. Hence, WC has been accepted as a better anthropometric in accessing central adiposity because it gives a better correlate of abdominal and visceral adiposity as WHR.

2.10.6.1 Waist circumference and Asian Indian

There are marked sex differences in the proportion of abdominal fat mass and for any accumulation of total body fat; males have twice as much abdominal fat as compared to pre-menopausal females. Also, different populations or ethnic groups have been shown to have marked differences in the risk of co-morbidities associated with abdominal fat accumulation (Shetty, 2000).

The level of risk associated with a particular waist circumference appears to vary with sex and ethnicity. Women have a relatively greater risk for cardiovascular disease at a lower cut-off (WHO, 2000[1]). In the WHO multinational monitoring of trends and determinants of cardiovascular disease (MONICA) project considerable variation in waist circumference (13cm to 15cm) among populations was noted (Molarius et al, 1999). The various waist circumference cut-off on basis of ethnicity are given in table 2.10.6.1

Table 2.10.6.1 Cut-off points for waist circumference varying with ethnicity

Ethnicity	Waist circumference cut-off (cm)		Reference
	Male	**Females**	
Caucasians	≥ 102	≥ 88	WHO, 2000[1]
Asians	≥ 90	≥ 80	WHO, 2000[2]
Japanese	> 85	> 90	Matsuzawa et al, 2000

Thus, the data indicates that cut-off points for WC vary among different populations. Nevertheless, it is clear that BMI or WC show a continuous linear relations with risk factors and clustering of risk factors, without any obvious breakpoint or threshold value, and a substantial overlap existed in the distribution curve of BMI and WC for populations with or without certain risk factors. Supplementation with body circumferences and body fat percent data allows for a more comprehensive overview with respect to status of obesity in a population (Zhou 2002). Population based epidemiological studies identified truncal obesity as risk factor for metabolic syndrome. Thereofre, a waist circumference value of ≥ 72 cm was considered as action level-I for Asians to identify metabolic risk (Gupta et al, 2009; Misra et al, 2009).

2.10.6.2 Waist stature ratio (WSR)

It is a novel and a simple index. It has only one variable as compared to WHR. In WSR, WC (variable) reflects abdominal obesity and height is constant in adults and can be used to compensate for variations in frame size (Hsieh et al, 2003).

WSR has been found to correspond better to metabolic risk than BMI, WC, WHR or skin fold measures in both men and women as well as those who are overweight and those of normal weight, who nevertheless face higher metabolic risks from central fat distribution (Hsieh and Yoshinga, 1995; Hsieh et al, 2000).

Garnett et al (2008) reported that the waist to height ratio cut-point of 0.5 estimated CVD risk clustering to a similar extent to sex and age adjusted cut points for waist circumference and BMI in Australian adults. People with excess central obesity (WSR ≥ 0.5) were 11 times (OR 11.4, $p<0.001$), more likely to have CVD risk clustering compared to those who did not have excess central adiposity.

Hsieh et al, 2003 in their study of Japanese men (n=6141) and women (n=2137) concluded that a waist/height cut-point ≥ 0.5 is most appropriate for signalling metabolic risk in the normal weight as well as overweight subjects.

Ashwell and Hsieh, 2005 gave six reasons for the use of waist to height ratio as a global indicator for health risks of obesity. Researchers suggest a simple, easily understood message for all i.e "keep your WC to less than half your height" (Garnett et al, 2008; Ashwell and Hsieh, 2005).

2.10.6.3 Fat mass index (FMI) and Fat free mass index (FFMI)

Weight comprises of both the FFM and FM and both these components can vary between individuals (Wells et al, 2002 Eto et al, 2004). The major shortcoming of

BMI is that the actual composition of body weight is not taken into account: excess body weight may be due to adipose tissue or muscle hypertrophy, both of which will be judged as excess mass (Schutz et al, 2002; Nakao and Komiya, 2003; Eto et al, 2004). On the other hand, a deficit of BMI may be due to FFM deficit (Sarcopenia) or a mobilization of adipose tissue or both combined (Herber et al, 1996).

Traditionally, fat mass has been normalized by expressing it as a percentage of body weight, whereas FFM tends to be expressed in absolute units, unadjusted for body size (Kyle et al, 2002). Since FFM and FM change with height, weight and age, it is difficult to determine whether individual subjects have a low or high FFM or FM (Kyle et al, 2003). The use of FFM in absolute terms complicates the interpretation because FFM is closely related to height and decreases with advancing age. Van Itallie et al (1990) demonstrated that stature explained 45% variance in FFM and 2% variance in FM. The use of percentage FM does not adequately reflect nutritional status because FFM automatically decreases in proportion to percentage FM increase (Kyle et al, 2003). This is undesirable as then a healthy and well nourished young individual can have values for these constituents that are virtually the same as those for similarly aged but taller individual who suffers from protein energy malnutrition (PEM) (Van Itallie et al, 1990). Also, two individuals with identical height and identical fat mass can have different body fat percentage because of the difference in their FFM content (Wells and Cole, 2002).

One potentially useful way to escape from the difficulties in interpreting data introduced by expressing FFM and FM as absolute values or percentages of body mass is to describe these components in terms of weight normalized for stature (Van Itallie, 1990). One such approach is to adjust body mass for stature and then separate this adjusted body mass into its FFM and FM components.

$$\textbf{BMI} = \frac{\text{Body Mass (Kg)}}{\text{Square of Height (m)}^2} = \frac{\text{FFM (Kg)}}{\text{Square of Height (m)}^2} + \frac{\text{FM (Kg)}}{\text{Square of Height (m)}^2}$$

$$\{\text{i.e. BMI (Kg/m}^2) = \text{FFMI (Kg/m}^2) + \text{FMI (Kg/m}^2)\}$$

The two indices i.e. FFMI and FMI are both discreet and adjusted for body size (Van Itallie, 1990).

The concept of FFMI and FMI have been previously described in adults and elderly subjects, as an indicator of nutritional status (Barlett et al, 1991) as well as in chronic obstructive pulmonary disease patients (Baaarends et al, 1997). They are easy to calculate and have the advantage of being expressed in common units of Kg/m^2 (Nakao and Komiya, 2003). Just as BMI is useful in evaluating the excess or deficit in body weight of individuals of different height, the FFMI and FMI are potentially useful in evaluating body composition parameters by effectively eliminating differences in FFM and FM associated with height (Kyle et al, 2003; Eto et al, 2004). Height independent body composition parameters like FFMI and FMI allow height independent interpretation of nutritional status, comparison of results between studies, and the development of body composition percentile tables (Kyle et al, 2003). Various studies in different parts of the world concluded that FMI and FFMI have higher levels of sensitivity than BMI in predicting obesity (Eto et al, 2004; Nakao and Komiya, 2003 and Kyle et al, 2003).

A study on Europeans in both men and women (15-98 years old) by Kyle et al (2003) represented FFMI and FMI values corresponding to low, normal, overweight and obese BMI. It was concluded that BMI alone is not sufficient in providing information on respective contribution of FFM or FM to body weight.

Uses of FMI and FFMI

FMI and FFMI can be used in a number of situations (Kyle et al, 2003) –

- They allow the tracking of the effects of illness, treatment, or aging in individuals and in groups because they can be interpreted as absolute values or by classifying individuals as normal or abnormal.
- FFMI also permits one to determine whether lower FFM with age is due to shorter height in older subjects or due to changes in body composition.
- FFMI and FMI also identify individuals with excess muscle mass but without excess body fat.

2.11 FACTORS AFFECTING WEIGHT STATUS

2.11.1 Age

WHO (2003) in its report on diet, nutrition and prevention of chronic diseases laid emphasis on adult years because it is the time period during which most chronic diseases are expressed as well as a critical time for preventive reduction of risk factors and for increasing effective treatment.

Wasuja and Siddhu (2002) reported significant positive association between weight and age ($r = +0.85$; $p<0.001$) in affluent women of Delhi till 60 years of age.

Also, Sternfeld et al (2004 observed a mean weight gain of 2.1 Kg over a period of three years in the study of women's health across the nation.

Body weight of women increases during early and middle adulthood (Stbye et al, 2011). Similar findings were reported by Agrawal and Mishra (2004) in their study on overweight and obese women in North India.

2.11.2 Weight status of parents

Various research studies have pointed towards the fact that obesity can be inherited. Lake et al (1997) concluded that the possibility of a child becoming an obese adult is markedly increased if both of his or her parents are obese. Rahilly and Farooqi (2006) in their study on genetics of obesity concluded that body mass index is a highly heritable trait. According to them, obesity in general population is largely due to mutation, which disrupts the function of hypothalamic integrative centers and results in increased food intake. Many of the hormonal and neural factors involved in normal weight regulations are determined genetically. These include the short and long term signals that determine satiety and feeding activity. Small defects in their expression or interaction could contribute significantly to weight gain. Also, the number and size of fat cells, regional distribution of body fat and RMR are influenced by genes (Prentice, 2005). Also, obesity during pregnancy has not been recognized to have a long term adverse affect on weight status of the offspring (Drake and Reynolds, 2010).

Kumanyika (2007) in her editorial wrote that obesity is an epidemic which is generally susceptible and is being transmitted through families to communities to whole society.

2.11.3 Parity

Studies support a positive association between parity and overweight among high income group of developing countries (Kim et al, 2007). Olson et al (2003) explained that cumulative cycle of post partum weight retention, as the mechanism by which parity leads to overweight.

2.11.4 Diet

Diet and nutrition are important factors in the promotion and maintenance of good health throughout the entire life cycle, and have well established role as determinants of non-communicable diseases including obesity and cardiovascular diseases.

Since the second half of the 20th century, great changes have swept the entire world, including major modifications in the diet, first in industrial regions and more recently in developing countries. It has resulted in a nutrition transition (Popkin, 2001; Popkin, 2002; Shetty, 2002).

The nutrition transition is characterized by unhealthy quantitative and qualitative shifts towards energy dense foods (sugar, fat, refined and processed foods, more foods of animal origin and alcohol) and reduced intake of fruits, vegetables, complex carbohydrates and fiber in the diet. Errors in eating pattern (irregular eating, skipping meals, night eating, overeating, etc) as well as lifestyle changes that reflect reduced physical activity at work and leisure further compound the problem (Popkin, 2001; Kanazawa et al, 2002; WHO, 2003). Nowdays, fast foods and high calorie snacks are replacing the other types of healthy foods resulting in obesity (Tiwari and Sankhala, 2007). The combination of changes in eating habits and sedentary lifestyles has contributed to the prevalence of overweight and obesity in the society. The increased consumption of foods with higher energy content, like those found in convenience meals, cause changes in the human organisms appetite control and contribute to the conditions of overweight an obesity (Prentice and Jebb, 2001; Martin et al, 2008).

Loren et al (2005) have explained how this nutrition transition towards a more westernized diet has led to fundamental alterations in the seven crucial nutritional characteristics – Glycemic Load, Fatty Acid Composition, Marco-nutrient Composition, Micro-nutrient Density, Acid Base Balance, Sodium Potassium Ratio and Fiber Content.

In a study by Kerver at al (2003) a dietary pattern was identified which was a predictor of CVD risk. This pattern was characterized by high intake of processed foods, eggs, red meats and high fat dairy products.

The global availability of cheap vegetable oils and fats has also contributed to the greatly increased fat consumption among developing countries (WHO, 2003). Yoo et al (2004) reported that low fruit and vegetable consumption and high sweetened beverage consumption are independently associated with prevalence of metabolic syndrome.

2.11.5 Energy expenditure and physical activity

Energy expenditure has an important role in controlling weight status. The difference between lean and obese subjects can be due to the difference in their energy expenditure pattern. It has been suggested that obese may be more energy efficient, i.e. they require fewer calories per unit of metabolically active body mass to maintain weight (Weinsier et al, 2002).

The 24 hour energy expenditure is composed of four components, the sleeping metabolic rate, the energy cost of arousal, the thermic effect of food (TEF) and energy cost of physical activity (Levine and Kotz, 2005). The first two components together form the basal metabolic rate (BMR).

2.11.5.1 Basal metabolic rate (BMR)

It is the largest component of energy expenditure, i.e. it accounts for 60%-75% of daily energy expenditure. Therefore, small deficits or excesses in BMR can add up to a large number of calories overtime (Ravussin and Bogardus, 1989; Dulloo and Schutz, 2005). BMR is influenced by various factors, like –

- Body size – people with greater surface area have higher metabolic rate (Frary and Johnson, 2008).

- Body composition – fat free mass (FFM), the metabolically active tissue in the body is a predictor of BMR. FFM contributes to approximately 80% of variance in BMR. In contrast the contribution of adipose tissue to BMR is small (Illner, 2000; Bosy-Westphal, 2004).

- Age – since BMR is determined by FFM, therefore BMR is highest during periods of rapid growth, chiefly during the first and second years of life (Butte, 2000). As a child grown older, the caloric requirement for growth is reduced to about 1% of total energy requirement (Roberts and Young, 1988). After early adulthood, there is a decline in BMR by 1-2% per kilogram of FFM per decade (Keys, 1973). Exercise can help maintain a higher lean body mass and thus a higher BMR (Dolezar and Potteiger, 1998).

- Sex – sex difference in metabolic rate are primarily attributable to differences in body size and composition (Frary and Johnson, 2008). However, day to day intra-individual variability in BMR is lower in men (coefficient of variation of 1-3%), but is larger in women because of changes in BMR over the menstrual cycle (Dulloo and Schutz, 2005).

- Genetic factor – genetic factor affects BMR as demonstrated by Ravussin and Bogardus (1989) that BMR varied upto ± 10% between individuals of the same age, gender, body weight and FFM.

- Others factors – other factors like hormonal status can affect metabolic rate in people with endocrine disorders or during periods of emotional excitement/stress when epinephrine is released (Frary and Johnson, 2008). Even the consumption of caffeine, nicotine and alcohol stimulate the metabolic rate (Compher, 2006). BMR is also affected by extremes in environmental temperature.

2.11.5.2 Thermic Effect of Food (TEF)

Thermic effect of food (TEF) is the increase in energy expenditure associated with the consumption of food. It accounts for almost 10% of total energy expenditure (TEE) (Dulloo and Schutz, 2005).

TEF plays an important role in weight management because it varies with the composition of the diet (Prentice, 1995). TEF is greater after consumption of carbohydrate and protein as compared to fat. Fat is metabolized efficiently with only 4% wastage as compared to 25% wastage when carbohydrate is converted to fat for storage. Farschi et al (2004) observed that TEF response was higher for women who followed a regular eating schedule as compared to those who ate irregularly.

2.11.5.3 Physical activity

It is most variable component of energy expenditure. Human physical activity is a complex behavior that is influenced by personal motivation, health and mobility issues, genetic factors and the social and physical environment in which people live. These factors exert an influence on the propensity to engage in sedentary behaviors as well as in physical activity (Hamilton et al, 2007). However, being the key determinant of energy expenditure, physical activity is fundamental to energy balance and weight control. Increased mechanization with technological advancements has led to the evolution of energy saving obesogenic societies. There is a shift from physically active to sedentary occupations, less walking and cycling with more use of cars and labour saving devices at work and at home. Inactivity during leisure with rapid increase of television use is a clear trend, especially among urban residents (Shetty, 2002; WHO, 2003; Muntner et al, 2005).

Data from 212,021 adults from 51 countries, most of which were developing countries, in the World Heath Survey (2002-2003) showed that about 15% of men and 20% of women were at risk of chronic disease due to physical inactivity (Guthold et al, 2008). The prevalence of physical inactivity at less than the levels recommended for enhancing health was high in developing countries, ranging from 17% to 91% (Oldbridge, 2008).

Data from Sã o Paulo, Brazil indicate that 70-80% of the population is remarkably inactive (Matsudo et al, 2002). In Colombia, an estimated 7.6% of all cause mortality and 20.1% of mortality due to chronic diseases were attributed to physical inactivity, and an estimated 5% of the mortality due to chronic diseases were preventable, if physical inactivity was reduced by 30% (Lobelo et al, 2006).

Kanazawa et al, 2002 suggested that inactivity may be the main cause for the increased incidence of obesity in Japan. It has been established that physically passive behaviors are associated with elevated body fat percent and associated co-morbidities (Kurpad et al, 2007).

Physical activity refers to any bodily movement produced by skeletal muscles that results in energy expenditure (Tsintsifa et al, 2006).

Diet and exercise have complementary beneficial influences on reducing the risk of chronic diseases associated with obesity (Miller et al, 1990; Chaput et al, 2009).

May et al (2010) reported that an increase in physical activity was associated with a statistically significant lower gain in body weight and in waist circumference which was maintained during the following five years in a ten year Doetinchen Cohort Study.

Research studies have reported that the people who exercise regularly are more likely to adopt healthy eating patterns like limiting fat intake and having an adequate consumption of fruits and vegetables. Also, high aerobic fitness was associated with increased consumption of carbohydrates and decreased consumption of fat when compared with those in lower fitness categories (Tsintsifa et al, 2006; Armstrong et al, 1990; Titchenal, 1988).

In a STRRIDE (studies of targeted risk reduction interventions through defined exercise) – a randomized controlled clinical trial, it was observed that there was a clear dose response relationship between the amount of weekly exercise and amount of weight change. It was observed that modest amount of exercise (walking 30 min/d) can prevent weight gain with no changes in the diet (Slentz et al, 2004).

Summerbell et al (2009) concluded that baseline physical activity was, in general, not associated with subsequent weight gain but change in physical activity was related to concurrent weight change.

Regular physical activity is very important for everyone, especially people who are trying to lose weight or maintain a low body weight (Jakicic and Otto, 2005).

2.11.6 Body image and body dissatisfaction

Body image is the term that has come to be widely accepted "as the internal representation of your own outer appearance, your own unique perception of your body" (Thomson, 2011).

Modern western culture emphasizes thinness, denigrates excess weight, and stigmatizes obese individuals. Researches suggest that exposure to media images, which depicts the thin-ideal and beautiful women to be linked to body image disturbances and mood states in women (Grabe et al, 2008).

Schwartz and Brownell (2004) reported that obesity is linked with poor body image but not all obese persons suffer from this problem.

Body dissatisfaction can be defined as a perceptive component of body image, as a difference between ideal body weight and current body size (Thompson, 2011). Body dissatisfaction has been an issue not only for women who have eating disorders, but also for non clinical population as well, and to such an extent that many American psychologists consider it a normative aspect of any women's identity (Garner, 1997).

Lamb et al (1993) studied attitudes about body and level of body dissatisfaction in two groups of women – a group younger than 20y and one older than 40y. Both the groups showed body dissatisfaction, but it was higher among the younger group.

Ŝivert et al (2008) also reported that body dissatisfaction is present in women of all ages regardless of their marital status, level of education and profession. However, the level of dissatisfaction is lesser among older women.

2.11.7 Stress

Stress permeates to every age category being an unavoidable consequence of life in today's day and age. Stresses may be physical, mental or emotional, personal or occupational. These may include common daily stresses like work pressures and discord with friends or relatives, etc. Trauma, injury and surgery are also major stressors to the body. It is commonly believed that most people respond to stress by abnormal food behavior like reduction in eating or overeating (Schachter et al, 1972). Thus, some people lose weight while under stress and other become fat due to excessive calories contributed by and increased appetite.

Depression, which is more common in women than in men, has been associated with overeating and weight gain, both with respect to using food for comfort and because many any depressants cause weight gain (Gorman, 2006). Also, in a survey by Zellner et al (2006), more women than men reported overeating under stress.

In a sterling county study, it was reported that depression among obese subjects in a community sample tends to be more severe than among non-obese subject (Murphy et al, 2009).

2.12 GENDER RELATED DIFFERENCE IN OBESITY PREVENTION

Women on average are more interested in food and nutrition and eating healthier diets as compared to men. Nevertheless, obesity prevention is more difficult for women than men (Satia et al, 2005). Researchers argue that women have lower caloric requirements than men and therefore must consume less food then men if they are to remain in energy balance. However, this is particularly disadvantageous for women when eating out because restaurant and take home portion sizes have increased and are same for all customers whether male or female (Girois et al, 2001). This unwitting consumption of a few hundred extra kilocalories is more detrimental to energy balance for women than men because the amount of calories expended is proportional to body size and amount of lean tissue. In comparison to men women have a smaller body size and less lean tissue, which results in lower energy expenditure (AHA, 2008).

2.13 RATIONALE FOR THE STUDY

Looking at the role of Indian woman in this era we find that she has a three-dimensional role to play i.e.

Biological – which implies reproduction and lactation.

Social – which includes woman's domestic responsibilities.

Economic – her role as an income earner.

A woman is therefore subjected to different health stresses over a span of her life owing to her productive and reproductive roles (Lukmanji, 1992).

In India, women's health has not received the attention it deserves but lately body image has become important. There is an urge in the overweight/obese women to reduce weight and even the normal women want to look thin to become socially more acceptable. This has lead to the growth of number of health clinics claiming to reduce weight in a short span of time along with other health benefits.

Body weight status of Indian women is of concern because rapid economic changes have led to increased household income and ownership of consumer goods, more sedentary jobs and reduced domestic work burden and labour saving devices. Further, with a disadvantaged genetic phenotype, it predisposes them to conditions like type 2 diabetes and cardiovascular diseases (CVD), which have a direct relationship with overweight and obesity (Popkin, 1998; James et al, 2001; Misra et al, 2005). But within this same socio-economic group there are women with normal weight. Therefore an insight into the physical activity levels, dietary behaviour and social life of women who have maintained normal weight versus those who have gained weight (overweight/obese) in the age group of 25-45 years will help to understand the role of various parameters on their body weight status. Positive deviance factors, which contribute to maintenance of weight, need to be studied and well established. This in turn will help to formulate appropriate intervention by lifestyle modifications.

Increasing evidence shows that early developmental origin of adult disease is linked to both maternal undernutrition and over nutrition with adverse long-term consequences in terms of obesity, type 2 diabetes and cardiovascular disease among their offspring (Barker, 1992; Caballero, 2001; Osmani and Sen, 2003). Most of the data on trends of overweight and obesity in developing countries is coming from cross sectional surveys, -but there is still very little information on weight trends and physical activity level of adult woman in the reproductive age group. Therefore, there is necessity for population based assessment of the patterns, distribution and determinants of normal weight status among women of child bearing age.

BROAD OBJECTIVE

Therefore the present study aims at comparing the normo weight adult women in the reproductive age group belonging to urban upper middle and high income groups with those in overweight/obese group with respect to their physical activity, dietary behaviour, reproductive health variables and social factors. The specific objectives of the study are as follows:

SPECIFIC OBJECTIVES

1. To assess the weight status of urban women aged 25 to 45 years by anthropometry in order to classify normoweight and excess weight.
2. To estimate body composition of BMI categories.
3. To identify health profile and co-morbidities associated with weight.
4. To assess their physical activity pattern, dietary intake and energy status.
5. To identify dietary and lifestyle factors important for maintaining normal weight status.

3. METHODOLOGY

The present research endeavour was an attempt to understand the wide variety of factors associated with desirable body weight among adult urban affluent women in the reproductive age group. To get a better insight of the factors, energy intake (EI), energy expenditure (EE), dietary pattern and energy status as well as the physical activity pattern of the subjects were studied. Both qualitative and quantitative approaches were used to elicit the required information.

3.1 DESIGN OF THE STUDY

3.1.1 Locale of Investigation

The study was carried out in selected residential colonies of National Capital Territory (NCT) of Delhi. The colonies were selected on the basis of economic strata of the inhabitants to ensure a fair degree of homogeneity and similar living conditions. The study was conducted on women belonging to upper middle and high socio-economic strata. Affluent colonies from four zones of Delhi, i.e. North, South, East and West were selected as under:

(i)	South Zone	South Extension, Part-I and Part-II, New Delhi
(ii)	North Zone	Ashok Vihar, Phase – I, Delhi
(iii)	East Zone	UNESCO Apartments and Sri Ram Apartments both at Patparganj, Delhi
(iv)	West Zone	Printers Apartments, Rohini, Delhi

Criteria for selection of locale

- These areas had a well organized Residential Welfare Association (RWA). The members of these locale readily volunteered to participate in the study.
- They had a facility of a community hall/centre, where the investigator could

meet the study subjects.

- These societies were regularly conducting health camps/melas for their residents and the residents readily participated in these events.

3.1.2 Sample Size

The sample size was ascertained by keeping level of significance (α) = 0.05 and prevalence value of obesity (p)=0.6 on epistat statistical package and calculated. The detailed calculation of sample size estimation has been shown in **Annexure-1**.

The calculated value of the sample size was 369. The (p) value was based on the research data that there is 60% prevalence of overweight and obesity amongst urban healthy women in Delhi in the age group of 30 to 49 years (Wasuja & Siddhu, 2002).

3.1.3 Sample Selection

The sample comprises of urban upper middle and HSES women aged 25-45 years with parity. The sample has been selected through purposive sampling.

The subjects for the study were identified by holding a body composition camp in the selected residential areas with the help of the RWA. From the information obtained at the body composition camp a list of eligible women in the age group of 25-45 years was prepared. These women were contacted telephonically to seek their willingness for participating in the study. Those willing and wilfully consented to participate in the study were enlisted.

The purposive sample was selected after using the inclusion/exclusion criteria. The **inclusion** criteria for the study were as under:

- Woman should be belonging to upper middle or HSES ie house hold income $\geq$ Rs.9,60,000/- per annum (NCAER, 2006-2007)
- Woman should be in the reproductive age group
- Woman should be married and having atleast one living child
- Woman should be with BMI of $\geq$ 18.5 Kg/m^2

The **exclusion** criteria for the study were as under:

- Women belonging to LSES based on total income within selected colonies
- If she has had a hysterectomy or attained menopause
- If she was pregnant or nursing
- If BMI < 18.5 Kg/m^2

From these camps in six localities, 432 women were eligible, of which 387 consented. Therefore, the final study sample size was of 387 women.

The sample was categorized into four BMI categories, i.e. Normal (N), at risk of over weight/pre-overweight (PO), overweight (OW) and Obese (Ob) based on WHO 2004 classification for Asians, as presented in Table 3.1.3

Table 3.1.3 IOTF – Proposed classification of BMI categories for Asians (WHO, 2004)

BMI (Kg/m^2)	Classification
18.5 – 22.9	Normal (N)
23.0 – 24.9	At risk of overweight / pre-overweight (PO)
25.0 – 29.9	Overweight (OW)
≥ 30.0	Obese (Ob)

(WHO, 2004)

The basis for using this classification was that WHO Expert Consultation, in its Lancet publication in 2004, reported after a meta-analysis of population data from more than 10 countries, that the proportion of Asian people with a higher risk of type – 2 diabetes and cardio-vascular disease is substantial at BMIs lower than the existing

WHO cutoff point for overweight (≥ 25 Kg/m^2). This consultation also agreed that the WHO BMI cutoff points should be retained as International classification and suggested lower BMI action points of 23.0, 27.5, 32.5 and 37.5 Kg/m^2 for individual countries to define the cutoff points for increased risk for their populations and for reporting purposes, with a view to facilitate international comparisons (WHO, 2010).

3.1.4 Data Collection

The study was carried out in two phases:

Phase – I : Quantitative Data Collection

- Administration of questionnaire among the subjects
- Anthropometric measurements of subjects
- Body composition assessment
- Dietary intake
- Energy expenditure and physical activity.

Phase – II : Qualitative Data Collection

- Focus group discussion (FGD) for bringing out barriers and enhancers for weight loss and maintenance respectively.

3.2 RESEARCH DESIGN

The schematic representation of the research design of the study carried out in a sequential manner is presented in Fig. 3.2.1

Fig. 3.2.1 Research Design of the Study

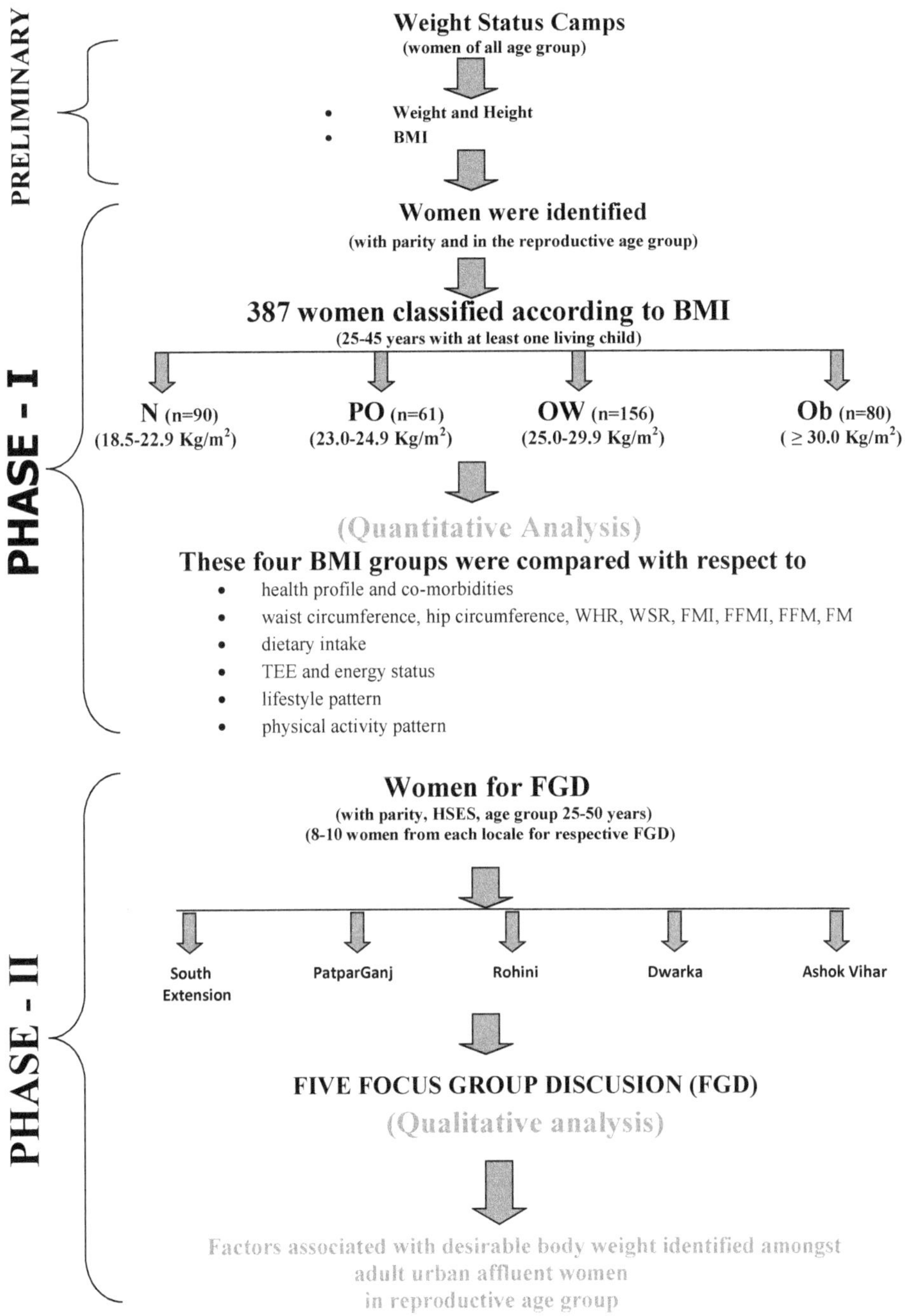

3.3 TOOLS AND TECHNIIQUES

The table 3.3 presents the summary of tools and techniques used in the present study for data collection.

Table 3.3 Summary of tools and techniques used for data collection

Sr. No.	Data Collected	Tools and Techniques
1	General Information	Oral Questionnaire
2	Anthropometric Measurements • Weight • Height • Circumference of waist & hip	Digital Weighing Scale Anthropometrical Rod PVC coated flexible fibre glass, measuring tape
3	Body Composition • Body Fat percent • Fat Mass • FFM • TBW	TBF – 300 Tanita Body Composition Analyser
4	Dietary Assessment	two 24 hour recall
5	Energy Expenditure Data • Basal Metabolic Rate • Total Day's Energy Expenditure	Prediction equation (ICMR 2010) Factorial Method (2 day's activity recall)
6	Identification of factors responsible for weight gain/loss and maintenance	Focus Group Discussion
7	Analysis • Anthropometric Data, Body Composition and Dietary Data • Nutrient Intake Data • Significance Test at $\alpha = 0.05$	Mean and S.D Diet Soft Chi-square test, ANOVA , Pearson Correlation, ROC curve and Binary logistic regression analysis

Phase-1 of the study

3.3.1 Phase – I : Quantitative data collection

For the present study four set of questionnaires were designed to elicit information on the following parameters:

- General information
- Health profile amd co-morbidities
- Diet history, dietary pattern and eating out pattern
- Daily activity pattern

The questionnaire on general information included questions on chronological age, marital status, educational qualification, family structure, number of family members, occupational status and income profile of the subjects.

Health profile included questions on co-mordidities present, type of treatment/medication or supplements used and the weight status of the parents. Also information related to self preceition of weight, weight gain/loss after pregnancy as well as per annum and information regarding reproductive health variables like age of onset of menarche, regularity of menstrual cycle, history of intake of oral contraceptives, etc., was obtained.

The questionnaire on diet history, dietary pattern and eating out pattern helped in eliciting information related to food habits, type of diet, fasting, overeating, eating in between meals, snacking pattern, dietary restrictions and especial diet during pregnancy and lactation, meal pattern, like and dislike, frequency of eating out, food preference while eating out and any specific modifications in diet.

The questionnaire on activity pattern included questions on activities being performed during the day along with the frequency of performing that activity. Also, questions pertaining to type of domestic help employed, time spent on house hold activities, sleeping, television viewing, recreational activities with children and choice of mode of transportation for commuting to neighbourhood places, use of stair case, travelling and activities while on holiday were asked.

The questionnaires were pre-tested on 10% of the proposed sample and were suitably modified according to the responses received. The final versions of the questionnaires are given in **Annexure – 2 (a) to Annexure – 2 (d).**

The questionnaires were filled by the subjects and were returned back when the investigator visited them for collecting information on dietary intake and activity pattern. Any unanswered question(s) was personally clarified by the investigator from the respondents either on telephone or during home visit. Prior consent from the respondents was taken and their convenient meeting time was fixed on telephone before visiting/meeting them. Most of the housewives preferred pre-lunch time between 10.30 a.m. and 2.00 p.m. when they were free from their morning chores. Whereas, the working mothers preferred meeting in their office during their free/leisure time mostly during lunch hours or they preferred clarifying on telephone.

3.3.2 Anthropometric Assessment

Anthropometric assessment was done during the weight status camps organized by the RWA in their community centre.

Anthropometry is the measurement of the body size, weight and proportions. Measurements obtained from anthropometry can be sensitive indicators of overall health and long term nutritional status. Anthropometric methods are also non-invasive, inexpensive and universally acceptable (Jellife et al, 1989). This is a fast method for nutritional assessment and results can be numerically graded. Anthropometry along with other components of nutritional assessment can evaluate under nutrition, over nutrition and can also be used as a basic plan to monitor the effect of nutritional interventions in people at nutritional risk (Baer and Harris, 1997).

3. METHODOLOGY

In the present study, anthropometric measures like weight, height, waist circumference and hip circumference were measured using standardized tools and techniques. All the measures were taken in duplicate.

Weight Weight is the key anthropometric measurement indicator of current nutritional status (Jellife et al, 1989). The relationship between body weight and mortality has been widely investigated with both lean and obese people showing an increased mortality (Jarrett et al, 1982; Wannamethee and Shaper, 1989, 1990; Calle et al, 2005).

A digital weighing scale with a sensitivity of 0.1 kg was used for recording weight. The balance was used because it is portable, light, easy to operate and convenient for field work (Gibson, 2005). The machine was calibrated with standard weights and accuracy was checked from time to time with a known weight of 20 kg. The subjects were weighed barefooted and with minimum clothing (Jellife et al, 1989).

Height was measured with the help of a anthropometrical rod which read upto a minimum of 0.1 cm. The subjects were made to stand barefoot on a flat surface with heels together, legs straight, arms by the side and shoulders relaxed. The head was positioned in the Frankfurt plane and the anthropometrical rod was placed behind the subjects so that the lower end was behind the heels and beam passed vertically between the buttocks touching the back of the head. The headpiece was lowered onto the crown of the head with sufficient pressure to compress the hair. The reading was taken at the eye level to the head piece (Gibson, 2005).

Body Mass Index (BMI) has been recognized as a simple, responsive and useful indicator of nutritional status of adults. It serves as an important and valuable tool for monitoring nutritional status of populations (Shetty, 1994). BMI is a most useful epidemiological tool in estimating the prevalence of obesity and chronic under nutrition and the increased risk of morbidity and mortality associated with these nutritional states (Shetty, 2003). It is one of best index for measuring nutritional status (Garrow and Webster, 1985; James et al, 1988; Naidu and Rao, 1994). A WHO sponsored expert consultation on obesity advocated the use of BMI to determine the weight status of individuals (WHO, 2000[2]).

The BMI is calculated as: BMI = weight (kg) / height $(m)^2$

International obesity task force (IOTF) proposed classification of BMI categories for Asians (WHO, 2004) has been used for determining the weight status of the subjects. The proposed classification has been given earlier in the table 3.1.3.

Waist to Hip Ratio (WHR) is a simple index of body fat distribution and provides an indication of the distribution of fat storage in the abdominal region. A high WHR is indicative of centripetal distribution of body fat. Abdominal adiposity has been shown to be associated with risk of overall mortality in many populations (Han et al, 1995; Okusun et al, 1998). WHR gives a measure of amount of abdominal fat which is a clinical correlate of metabolic disturbances and abdominal obesity (Ashwell et al 1985).

To calculate WHR, waist and hip circumference are required. A WHR of > 1.0 for men and > 0.85 for women was used as an indicator of abdominal obesity (Hodge et al, 1993; Shetty, 2000).

Waist Circumference also reflects the magnitude of abdominal adipose tissue deposited as well as the total fat mass and thereby complements BMI in the evaluation of obesity and measure of body fat distribution. In fact several studies have shown that it is superior to BMI in its association with CVD risk factors (Pouliot et al, 1994; Zhu et al, 2002). It reflects intra-abdominal and subcutaneous fat. The waist circumference of the overweight/obese subjects and normal weight subjects was measured to the nearest 0.1 cm, using a PVC coated non-stretchable fibreglass tape.

Waist circumference is measured midway between the tenth rib i.e., the lowest rib margin and the iliac crest in a horizontal plane. Each bony landmark is palpated and marked, and the midpoint determined with a tape measure and marked (WHO, 1995).

In obese subjects, it is difficult to palpate these bony landmarks therefore waist circumference is measured at the narrowest waist above the umbilicus (Wang et al, 2003).

The subject is made to stand comfortably with her weight evenly distributed on both feet and feet about 25-30 cm apart. The observer sits by the side of the subject and fits the tape snugly but not so tight as to compress the underlying soft tissues.

Asian Indians have smaller body size, excess body fat, truncal and abdominal adiposity but lower average waist circumference than white Caucasians (Misra and Vikram, 2004).

Modified waist circumference cut-offs for Asians i.e. > 90 cm in men and > 80 cm in women are being used instead of > 102 cm in men and > 88 cm in women (WHO, 2004; Misra et al, 2005).

Additionally, subjects with waist circumference $\geq$ 72 cm for women, which is considered as action level 1 for Asian Indian women was also taken into account. These subjects were advised to avoid weight gain, or told to lose weight, and maintain increased physical activity (Misra et al, 2006; Misra et al, 2009).

Hip Circumference is measured at the maximum protrusion of the buttocks. The subject is made to stand erect with arms at the sides and feet together. The investigator sits at the side of the subject so that the level of maximum extension of the buttocks can be seen, and places the tape measure around buttocks in a horizontal plane. The tape is snug against the skin but does not compress the soft tissues (WHO, 1995).

A WHR of > 1.0 for men and > 0.85 for women was used as an indicator of abdominal obesity (Hodge et al, 1993; Shetty, 2000).

A non-stretchable flexible PVC coated fibre glass tape with a sensitivity of 0.1 cm was used for measuring the hip circumference.

Waist stature ratio (WSR) is a novel and a simple index. It has only one variable as compared to WHR. In WSR, waist circumference (variable) reflects abdominal obesity and height is constant in adults and can be used to compensate for variations in frame size (Hsieh et al, 2003).

In order to calculate WSR, waist circumference and height measurement are required. In the present study WSR cut-off ≥ 0.5 has been used as a measure of central obesity (Hsieh et al, 2003; Ashwell and Hsieh, 2005; Garnett et al, 2008).

3.3.3 Body Composition

Body composition assessment was done during health camps organized by the RWA in their community centre.

Body composition analysis serves as an important measure for evaluating and monitoring nutritional status and health (Radley et al, 2003). Traditional methods like hydro-densitometry based on a 2-compartment model of body, i.e. fat and fat free mass (FFM) was a gold standard for measurement of body composition. Sometimes to increase the accuracy an independent estimate of total body water (TBW), under 3-compartment model can be used in conjunction with hydro-densitometry (Kurpad, 2003). Other newer techniques like DEXA that measures bone mineral content, under 4-compartment model can also further improve the precision. Further, magnetic resonance imaging, in vivo neutron activation analyses are some of the latest techniques with high precision and cost. However, study of these compartment models are difficult to apply in the field because of sophisticated equipment, large sample size and lack of cost effectiveness, alternately, BIA which is a non invasive and easily applied methodology has been developed for field use.

BIA is a relatively easy method for measuring TBW based on the measured resistance of the body to the passage of a small electric current that yields accurate results of resistance and therefore the impedance to current flow. These impedance values are used to calculate TBW (Kushner, 1992). Equations for predicating FFM and body fat using impedance with appropriate cross validation have been developed in adults by several authors abroad (Heitman, 1990; Deurenberg et al, 1991) and in Asian Indians (Kuriyan et al, 1998). Such equation tends to be specific to the populations for which they were developed and both age and ethnicity may be important predicators (Gallagher et al, 1996; Rush et al, 2003). For measurement of body fatness, bioelectrical impedance analysis (BIA) has a distinct advantage over BMI because it differentiates between fat and lean tissue whereas BMI does not.

Tanita Body Composition Analyzer (TBF-300) was used for measuring body composition. The device is based on the principles of bioelectrical impedance. Tanita utilizes patented "foot to foot" pressure contact electrode. A low energy, high frequency electrical signal (50 KHz, 500 micro-amps) is induced and measurement of the baseline resistance to the flow of electrical current in the body is made. This current is passed through the anterior electrode on the scale platform, and the voltage drop is then measured on posterior electrode. The resistance measurement relates directly to the volume of the conductor, which is used to determine total body water, lean body mass and fat mass. The visceral/abdominal fat is not determined separately.

The data for age, weight, sex, and standard/athlete body type was fed through a control box into Tanita body composition analyzer. The individual was then requested to step on the platform barefoot. The heels were placed directly on top of the posterior electrodes, while the front part of the foot was in contact with the anterior electrodes. Body fat mass (FM), fat free mass (FFM) and total body water (TBW), BMI and resistance was then displayed on printout.

3.3.3.1 Percentage Body Fat (PBF)

Though BMI is widely used to categorize overweight and obesity there is a large literature on relations between BMI and measures of body fat. Obesity can be defined as over storage of fat beyond 18%. Usually, body fat over 30% is considered obesity (Kanazawa et al, 2002). The upper limit of percent body fat is still a debatable issue. Different authors have arrived at different cut-offs of body fat percent for defining obesity. Hortobagyi et al (1994) have set 25% and 30 % as upper limits of body fat for males and females respectively. Siddhu (2004) recommended a cut-off of 35% body fat for obesity in young Indian women, which gave cutoff at BMI of 23 on ROC. In the study by Siddhu (2004) using 30% body fat as criterion, the sensitivity was 95.5% and specificity was 85.88 at BMI of 21 Kg/m^2. In another study by Dudeja et al (2001), on females aged 20-69 years, a lower cut-off value of BMI i.e 19.0 Kg/m^2 displayed the optimal sensitivity and specificity at 30% body fat as criterion. In a study by Misra et al (2003), using 30% body fat criterion, for female dyslipidaemic patients, a cut-off of 23 Kg/m^2 gave a sensitivity of 85.7% and specificity of 62.5%. Therefore, in the present study PBF value ≥ 30.0% and ≥ 35% was used to classify overweight and obesity, keeping in view the criteria given by Dudeja et al (2001) and Siddhu (2004) for North Indian women.

3.3.3.2 Fat Mass Index (FMI) and Fat Free Mass Index (FFMI)

Weight comprises of fat free mass (FFM) and fat mass (FM) and both these components can vary between individuals (Wells et al, 2002; Eto et al, 2004). The major shortcoming of the BMI is that the actual composition of the body weight is not taken into account. Excess body weight may be due to adipose tissue or muscle hypertrophy, both of which will be judged as excess mass (Schutz et al, 2002; Nakao and Komiya, 2003; Eto et al, 2004). On the other hand a deficit of BMI may be due to FFM deficit (Sarcopenia) or a mobilization of adipose tissue or both combined (Herber et al, 1996). Also fat mass and fat free mass have different health effects. When only BMI is used as a criterion of nutritional status, these divergent relationships can not be distinguished (Van Itallie,1990; Allison et al 1997; Heymsfield et al, 2005; Hull et al, 2011).

One potentially useful way to escape from the difficulties in interpreting data introduced by expressing FFM and FM as absolute values or percentages of body mass is to describe these components in terms of weight in Kg normalized for stature

(Van Itallie et al, 1990). The approach is to adjust body mass for stature and then separate this adjusted body mass into its FFM and FM components.

Therefore, the FFMI and FMI of the study subjects was calculated to have a better insight of the differences in the body composition of the women in the four BMI categories.

Since there are no published ranges of FFMI and FMI for Asian subjects, therefore in the present study, the values calculated for Caucasian women by Kyle et al (2003) have been used for comparison in the discussion (ref. 5.4). Kyle et al (2003) reported FFMI value of 14.6 Kg/m^2 to 16.8 Kg/m^2 and FMI value of 3.9 Kg/m^2 to 8.2 Kg/m^2 for Caucasian women fall within the normal BMI range.

3.3.4 Dietary intake assessment

The dietary intake data was planned to be obtained through 24 hour record for three days which included two working days and one holiday. The respondents were explained on how to keep an accurate record. Written instructions and a sample for recording of entries were provided with the dietary record form. The dietary record form is attached as **Annexure - 3**.

Common household measures like bowls (katori), glass, ladle (karchi) and spoons of different sizes were shown and respondents were asked to carefully record quantities of all foods and beverages consumed in these measures. The size of chapattis, thickness and consistency of foods consumed, type of fat and milk used, consumption of fruits, vegetables, beverages and other energy dense foods was also recorded.

However, at the end of the recording period, it was observed at the time of pre-testing most respondents were unable to record their intake and were returning their pro-forma incomplete. As a result dietary intake data was collected by two 24 hour recall technique. Also, subjects were asked questions on their daily consumption of milk, amount of fat consumed by the family in a month and whether they were using ghee/oil on chapatti/rice.

The data thereby obtained, was standardized by using known amounts of raw foods for cooking the reported food item to arrive at quantities of raw foods consumed. Some recipes were standardized in the Department of Foods and Nutrition, Lady Irwin College. The standardization of house hold measures of raw and cooked food stuffs at Lady Irwin College is provided in **Annexure – 4.** The intake of various food items and nutrients was computed for each day separately using computer software called "Diet-Soft" version 1.17 copyright, 2009, which uses the data base of raw foods given in the Nutritive Value of Indian Foods (ICMR, 1989).

3.3.5 Energy expenditure and activity pattern

Total Energy Expenditure (TEE) is defined as the average energy spent in a 24 hour period by an individual or by a group of individuals. By the definition itself, it reflects the average amount of energy spent on a typical day, but it is not the exact amount of energy spent each and every day (FAO/WHO/UNU, 2004).

Factorial Method

The FAO/WHO/UNU Expert Consultation on Energy Requirement (2004) has recommended to estimate TEE through factorial calculations that combined the time allotted to habitual activities and the energy cost (Physical Activity Ratio - PAR) of those activities. This committee also recommended use of Heart Rate Method (HRM) and DLW to compute TEE.

The most accurate field measure of energy expenditure is doubly labelled water (DLW). However, this approach has limited feasibility in terms of cost and use in studies of total energy expenditure only, as it does not describe the type or purpose of activity performed (Irwin et al, 2001; Lamonte and Ainsworth, 2001). Self reported physical activity records and surveys are low cost, relatively unobstructive method of assessing physical activity and energy expenditure in field setting and vary in terms of their format, mode of administration and degree of detailing habitual physical activity levels. Thus, they have a unique advantage of providing additional information on types of activity and time devoted by individuals to specific activities (Lamonte and Ainsworth, 2001; Conway et al, 2002).

In the present study, factorial method was used to compute TEE. The subjects were asked to maintain a minute to minute activity record on a pro-forma. The written instructions and a sample of recording was provided along with the pro-forma. The activity record pro forma is attached as **Annexure – 5.** The women were explained how to record their activities in the day in terms of nature, duration and posture by one day recall and were asked to record for the next two days. However, like dietary data, the subjects failed to record their activities minute to minute as had been explained to them. Therefore, the activity was recalled for two days along with the dietary recall. This data was used for calculating the total day's energy expenditure and energy balance as well as the time spent in various activities.

3.3.5.1 Method for calculating TEE by factorial method

- **Prediction of BMR** – For BMR prediction equations based on body weight, given by ICMR(2010) were used. The equations used in the study are as under:

Age (in years)	Prediction Equation for women
18-30	14.0 × B.W. (kg) + 471
30-60	8.3 × B.W. (kg) + 788

- **Activity Categorization** - As depicted by activity profile of the subjects, various activities performed during the day were matched with the activities for which PAR was available in FAO/WHO/UNU (2004).
- **Calculation of TEE (total energy expenditure)** – The energy costs of various activities expressed as a multiple of BMR, or PAR (physical activity ratio) as given by ICMR (2010), FAO/WHO/UNU (2004) were used. The activity cost are given in table 3.3.5.1

Table 3.3.5.1 PAR of activities of women	
Activity	**Average PAR (Females)**
Sleeping	1.0
Lying	1.2
Personal Care	2.3
Eating	1.6
Cooking	2.1
Office Work	1.5
General Household Work	2.8
Driving a Car	2.0
Sitting in a bus/car	1.2
Child Care	2.5
Walking at various paces	2.5
Chatting on the Phone	1.4
Playing cards / Board games	1.75
Leisure walk	2.5
Brisk walk	3.8
Light aerobic exercise	4.2
Watching T.V/Computer	1.4

Ref. FAO/WHO/UNU (2004)

The energy costs of these activities were calculated for each subject using the respective BMR values (Kcal/min) or (Kcal/hr). The total time (min/hr) spent on each activity category was calculated and was multiplied by the energy cost in order to obtain the energy expenditure (EE) during that activity. The sum total of EE on all activities gave TEE. Three day TEE was calculated and mean of two days was taken for the study.

- **Energy balance:** Energy balance (EB) was calculated by the following formula:

$$EB = TDEI - TEE$$

3.3.6. Phase – II: Qualitative data collection - Focus Group Discussion (FGD)

Quantitative techniques especially questionnaire surveys, used for eliciting information, only indicate what people know but give very little information on their claimed behaviour. In such a context, the use of qualitative techniques like FGDs is useful. The focus groups usually constitute a group of six to eight people, selected for their homogeneity on some factor important for research (Rao et al, 2008).

In the present study FGD technique was used to assess the perceived factors of weight gain and weight maintenance amongst women of the reproductive age group belonging to upper middle and HSES for the first time for evolving useful strategies.

For the present study, five FGD's were conducted in five different localities in Delhi, selected in phase-I, namely

(i) C – Block South Extension, Part -2, New Delhi;
(ii) UNESCO Apartments, Patparganj, New Delhi;
(iii) Printers Apartments, Rohini, Delhi;
(iv) IB Block, Ashok Vihar, Phase-I, Delhi; and
(v) Surya Cooperative Society, Dwarka, New Delhi.

Women drawn from all walks of life, including professional working women, non-professional working women and mothers who were homemakers with desirable body weight and overweight in the age group of 25 to 50 years participated in focus group discussion (FGD). In each of the five discussions 8 to 10 women participated, a number considered optimal for effective focus group communication (RHRC, 2004). The women were provided with information about the date and time of their focus group discussion. The location for the discussion was a community facility in the locality or the Housing Complex.

The sample for FGD was contacted through Residential Welfare Association (RWA). The telephone numbers were obtained through the RWA,s directory available at the Residential Welfare Office. During the telephonic conversation information regarding socio-demographic and health related information, including age, weight and height was obtained.

For use during the sessions, a list of open ended theme questions were developed to gather specific information and facilitate discussions concerning weight management and factors contributing to its success or failure. The theme/research questions were as follows:

(i) Is your body weight a cause of concern?
(ii) What reasons would you give for your present body weight status?
(iii) What methods you have adopted to lose/maintain your body weight?
(iv) Which methods worked best?
(v) Which methods did not show the results?
(vi) What is the contribution of your family members in your pursuit for desirable body weight?
(vii) What is the role of your neighborhood in maintaining weight?
(viii) How do you like to spend your leisure time?
(ix) Why is it difficult to lose weight?
(x) What is one burning comment or piece of information that you want to add, which I missed out?

The FGDs were conducted by a moderator and an observer (notes taker), who had been trained to conduct the FGD in a standardized way.

The women were seated in a semi-circle with the moderator in the centre. The FGDs were conducted in Hindi and English. The discussions were audio-taped, with the consent of the participants. The recordings were transcribed on the same day and analysed for responses.

3.3.7. Data Analysis

The collected quantitative data was consolidated and systematically tabulated.

- The BMI was calculated and using WHO (2004) cut-off points for Asians, the subjects were divided into four weight categories.

- The data obtained from the interview schedule cum questionnaire was consolidated systematically on MS-Excel and converted into frequencies and percentages to facilitate analysis of results. Results from four BMI categories were statistically compared using Chi-square test. The level of significance was calculated at (p=0.05).

- The data on age, height, weight, waist circumference, hip circumference, WHR, PBF, FFM, FM, FFMI, FMI and TBW was tabulated and represented as mean ± SD along with the range for each parameter. The mean values were statistically compared using ANOVA and post hoc test between four BMI categories.

- WHR was calculated and a value >0.85 was indicative of abdominal fat accumulation (WHO, 2000) for adult females. However, waist circumference is the preferred measure of abdominal obesity compared to WHR (WHO, 1998). A cut-off ≥80.0 cm waist circumference (WHO, 2004) was considered as abdominal obesity in adult females. Also, a cut off ≥ 72.0 cm was considered as action level - 1 for Asian Indian women (Misra et al, 2009).
- WSR was calculated and a value ≥0.05 was indicative of greater metabolic risk (Hsieh et al, 2003; Garnett et al, 2008).

- PBF cut off ≥30.0% and ≥35.0% was indicative of overweight and obesity respectively (Dudeja et al, 2001; Siddhu, 2004).

- FFMI and FMI values were compared with values for Caucasian women (Kyle, 2003).
- The nutrient content of the food intake was calculated using Diet Soft software, 2009. The intake of energy, protein, fat and other nutrients was represented as mean ± SD and compared with the respective RDA (ICMR, 2010 and ICMR, 1990).
- Correlation of sleep time, exercise time, sitting time and television viewing time with BMI was derived using Pearson Correlation (r).
- ROC curve was plotted to derive the cutoff of PAL for urban affluent Indian women (25-45 years).
- Binary logistic regression analysis was used to derive the final determining factors associated with normal weight status of women.
- The recorded discussions of the focus group were transcribed by the moderator on the same day after the discussion using the notes taken by the observer to supplement the tape recordings. The Hindi scripts were quoted verbatim in the text. The reports were interpreted on the basis of the theme questions and the factors associated with weight status were identified and highlighted.

Ethical clearance

Due ethical clearance for the study was taken from the Institutional Ethics Committee, Lady Irwin College, University of Delhi, New Delhi. The ethical clearance certificate is attached as **Annexure – 6.**

As a token of appreciation for participation in the body composition camp, all the participants were given a booklet titled "watch your weight and waist", which contained useful information on weight management. The booklet has been attached as **Annexure – 7.**

4. RESULTS

In the present study, the possible factors associated with desirable body weight among adult urban affluent women in the reproductive age group were investigated. The findings of the study have been presented under the following heads:

4.1 General Information / Background Information
4.2 Health profile and co-morbidities
4.3 Diet history
4.4 Dietary pattern
4.5 Eating out pattern
4.6 Activity pattern
4.7 Anthropometric indicators: weight status of 25-45 year women
4.8 Body composition parameters
4.9 Dietary intake
4.10 Energy expenditure and Energy status
4.11 Determinants of desirable body weight (quantitative data)
4.12 Determinants of desirable body weight (qualitative data): Focus Group Discussion - FGD

The study is divided in two phases:

- **Phase I – Quantitative Analysis:** study of women 25 – 45 year with respect to factors affecting weights status.
- **Phase II – Qualitative Analysis:** focus group discussion with respect to factors effecting weight status.

The sample comprised of 387 married women in the age group of 25 – 45 years with atleast one living child. Since the objective of the study was to identify factors associated with desirable body weight, the entire sample was divided into BMI categories on the basis of classification for Asians (WHO, 2004) into normal (N) (n=90), at risk/pre-overweight (PO) (n=61), overweight (OW) (n=156) and obese (Ob) (n=80). All the parameters were studied in these four categories.

4.1 GENERAL INFORMATION/SOCIO-DEMOGRAPHIC PROFILE

The data focused on age profile, educational level, work status, occupation, marital status, religion, type of family and economic status of the subjects. The details are presented in table 4.1.1 to 4.1.9.

4.1.1 Age profile

The age profile of the women in the 4 BMI categories has been given in Table 4.4.1 (a). The data revealed that majority of women were falling in two age categories of 30 years – 34.9 years (n=146; 37.8%) and 35 years – 39.9 years (n=124; 32.0%).

Table 4.1.1 (a) - Age distribution of the subjects in the four BMI categories; (n=387) ; % (n)

Age Category	N (n=90)	PO (n=61)	OW (n=156)	Ob (n=80)	% Total (n=387)	P – value
25 – 29.9 years	46.4(13)	3.6 (1)	42.9(12)	7.1(2)	7.2 (28)	<0.001(S)
30 – 34.9 years	22.6(33)	24.7(36)	29.5(43)	23.3(34)	37.7 (146)	
35 – 39.9 years	14.5(18)	12.9(16)	58.1(72)	14.5(18)	32.0 (124)	
40 – 45 years	29.2(26)	9.0(8)	32.6(29)	29.9(26)	23.1 (89)	

Parentheses indicate number of subjects.
The level of significance for Chi-square was taken as p<0.05); (S) indicates Significant.

Also, 23.0% were in 40-45 years and 7.2% were in 25-29.9 years. In the youngest age category, the highest number of subjects belonged to N, whereas in subsequent age categories subjects belonging to OW were highest. The distribution of subjects in the four BMI categories with respect to age categories was significantly different (p<0.001). Overweight/obesity increased with age as can be seen from the data on mean age of subjects in table 4.1.1 (b). The mean age of subjects in Ob, PO and OW was significantly higher (p=0.001) as compared to N. Thus, increasing age is a significant factor affecting weight status of subjects in the present study.

Table 4.1.1 (b) - Mean age of women in the four BMI categories; (n=387) (mean ± SD with range)						
	N (n=90)	PO (n=61)	OW (n=156)	Ob (n=80)	Total (n=387)	P – value
Mean age (Years)	34.6 ± 5.27 (25-45)	37.2 ± 5.01 (27-45)	37.0 ± 5.16 (25-45)	37.4 ± 5.18 (25-45)	36.5 ± 5.26 (25-45)	0.001(S)

The level of significance for ANOVA was taken as $p<0.05$; (S) indicates Significant.

4.1.2 Educational status of women

Since the study sample belonged to affluent families the educational status of the women revealed that only 2.6 %(n=10) of the women were less than graduate whereas majority of them had attained graduate (36.2%; n=140) and post graduate degrees (30.2%; n=117) as shown in Table 4.1.2. Also nearly 30 % (n=114) of the women had attained professional degrees. Apart from these 1.5% had obtained other qualifications besides graduation like M.Phil, Ph.D, Nursery teacher training, computer courses etc. Further it was observed that in the graduate category highest (32.1%; n=45) were in OW. Those who were not graduate was a very small sample (n=10) and all were OW. In the post graduate category highest (29.9%; n=35) were in Ob category. In the professional education category highest (57.9%; n=66) women were in OW.

Table 4.1.2 - Educational qualification of the subjects in the four BMI categories; (n=387) ; % (n)

Qualification	N (n=90)	PO (n=61)	OW (n=156)	Ob (n=80)	% Total (n=387)	P – value
< Graduation	0	0	100(10)	0	2.6 (10)	<0.001 S)
Graduation	27.1(38)	15.7(22)	32.1(45)	25(35)	36.2 (140)	
Post- Graduation	24.8(29)	19.7(23)	25.6(30)	29.9(35)	30.2 (117)	
Professional	20.2(23)	13.2(15)	57.9(66)	8.8(10)	29.4 (114)	
Any other	0	16.7(1)	83.3(5)	0	1.6 (6)	

Parentheses indicate number of subjects.
The level of significance for Chi-square was taken as $p<0.05$; (S) indicates Significant.

4.1.3 Work Status

When the women in the study sample were categorized as gainfully employed and not gainfully employed, they were almost equal in number. The data on work status has been given in Table 4.1.3 (a) and (b). It was observed that 43.2% (n=80) of the women in the gainfully employed group were in the OW category, followed by 22.7% (42) in Ob, 21.6%.

Whereas in the not gainfully employed group, 24.8% (n=50) women were in N, which was similar to gainfully employed (21.6%). But 37.6% (n=76) in OW and 18.8% (n=38) in Ob category.

There was no significant (p=0.225) difference among the four BMI categories with respect to the work status. However, in the gainfully employed group, significantly (p=.001) higher number of women were teachers as compared to other occupation choices.

Table 4.1.3 (a) - Work status of the women in the four BMI categories; (n=387) ; % (n)

Work Status	N (n=90)	PO (n=61)	OW (n=156)	Ob (n=80)	% Total (n=387)	P – value
Gainfully employed	21.6(40)	12.4(23)	43.2(80)	22.7(42)	47.8 (185)	0.225 (NS)
Not gainfully employed	24.8(50)	18.8(38)	37.6(76)	18.8(38)	52.2 (202)	

Parentheses indicate number of subjects.
The level of significance for Chi-square was taken as p<0.05; (NS) indicates Not Significant.

Table 4.1.3 (b) - Occupation of the women in the four BMI categories; (n=185) ; % (n)

Occupation	N (n=40)	PO (n=23)	OW (n=80)	Ob (n=42)	% Total (n=185)	P – value
Teacher	21.4(21)	10.2 (10)	47.9(47)	20.4(20)	53.0 (98)	0.001 (S)
Doctor	52.6(10)	15.8(3)	0	31.6(6)	10.4 (19)	
Any other	13.2(9)	14.7(10)	48.5(33)	23.5(16)	17.6 (68)	

Parentheses indicate number of subjects.
The level of significance for Chi-square was taken as p<0.05); (S) indicates Significant.

4.1.4 Number of children

The transition of society towards fewer children was quite evident. More than 50% of the women had just one child. The results have been tabulated in Table 4.1.4. The data revealed that significantly higher (p=0.001) number of women belonging to OW (43.2%) and Ob (23.0%) had two children as compared to N (17.5%) and PO (16.4%). In the present study, number of children was a significant factor affecting the weight status of the subjects.

Table 4.1.4 - Number of children of the women in the four BMI categories; (n=387) ; % (n)

Number of Children		N (n=90)	PO (n=61)	OW (n=156)	Ob (n=80)	% Total (n=387)	P – value
1 (one)	% in sample	28.4(58)	15.2(31)	37.8(77)	18.6(38)	52.7 (204)	0.001 (S
	% within group	64.4 (58)	50.8 (31)	49.4 (77)	47.5 (38)		
2 (two)	% in sample	17.5(32)	16.4(30)	43.2(79)	23.0(42)	47.3 (183)	
	% within group	35.6 (32)	49.2 (30)	50.6 (79)	52.5 (42)		

Parentheses indicate number of subjects.
The level of significance for Chi-square was taken as $p<0.05$); (S) indicates Significant.

4.1.5 Type of family

In the present study, women were grouped vis a vis type of family under two heads – joint family and nuclear family. Family set up consisting of husband, wife and children was termed as nuclear family, and set up other than nuclear family was termed joint family. Out of the total sample, 52.2% were living in a joint set up and 47.8% in a nuclear set up as shown in Table 4.1.5.

Table 4.1.5 - Type of family of the women in the four BMI categories; (n=387) ; % (n)

Type of family		N (n=90)	PO (n=61)	OW (n=156)	Ob (n=80)	% Total (n=387)	P – value
Nuclear	% in sample	23.2(43)	22.7(42)	34.1(63)	20.0(37)	47.8 (185)	0.002 (S)
	% within group	47.8 (43)	68.9 (42)	40.4 (63)	46.3 (37)		
Joint	% in sample	23.3(47)	9.4(19)	46.0(93)	21.3(43)	52.2 (202)	
	% within group	52.2 (47)	31.1 (19)	59.6 (93)	53.7 (43)		

Parentheses indicate number of subjects.
The level of significance for Chi-square was taken as $p<0.05$); (S) indicates Significant.

This is in contrast to the growing belief that the majority of the urban families are staying in nuclear setup. In the nuclear group, highest i.e. 34.1% (n=63) of women belonged to the OW category and N, PO and Ob were equally distributed. In the joint family group, highest i.e (46.0%; n=93) women were in the OW and lowest number in PO (21.3%). The within group analysis revealed that almost 60% of OW and 54% of Ob women were living in a joint family as compared to 52.2% of N and 31.1% of PO. The family type has a significant (p=0.002) effect on weight status.

4.1.6 Size of family

The table 4.1.6 (a) depicts the number of family members of the subjects in the four BMI categories. It was observed that 24.8% (n=96) of the sample had three members in their family, 25.3% (n=98) had four, 22.7% (n=88) had five and 25.1% (n=97) had more than six members in their family. However, significantly higher (p=0.001) percentage of women belonging to OW (50.0%) reported having five family members as compared to women in other three categories.

Table 4.1.6 (a) - Number of family members of the women in the four BMI categories; (n=387) ; % (n)

Number of family members	N (n=90)	PO (n=61)	OW (n=156)	Ob (n=80)	% Total (n=387)	P – value
Two (2)	0	0	100.0(8)	0	2.1 (8)	0.001 (S)
Three (3)	27.1(26)	24.0(23)	30.2(29)	18.8(18)	24.8 (96)	
Four (4)	17.3(17)	22.4(22)	36.7(36)	23.5(23)	25.3 (98)	
Five (5)	17.0(15)	12.5(11)	50.0(44)	20.5(18)	22.7 (88)	
≥ Six (6)	32.9 (32)	5.2 (5)	40.2 (39)	21.7 (21)	25.1 (97)	

Parentheses indicate number of subjects.
The level of significance for Chi-square was taken as $p<0.05$); (S) indicates Significant.

The mean number of family members in the four categories has been given in Table 4.1.6 (b). The data revealed that the highest mean number of family members belonged to N and lowest to PO.

The four BMI categories differed significantly (p=0.001) with respect to the size of the family.

Table 4.1.6 (b) - Mean number of family members of the women in the four BMI categories; (n=387) (mean ± SD with range)						
Mean number of family members	N (n=90)	PO (n=61)	OW (n=156)	Ob (n=80)	Total (n=387)	P – value
Mean	5.6 ± 3.3 (3-16)	3.97 ± 0.95 (3-6)	4.48 ± 1.6 (2-9)	5.12 ± 2.1 (3-9)	4.92 ± 2.3 (2-16)	<0.001 (S)
The level of significance for ANOVA was taken as p<0.05; (S) indicates Significant.						

4.1.7 Economic status

The subjects in the present study belonged to upper middle and high income group. The data of the family income, total number of earning members and per capita availability indicated that income was not a limiting factor.

The data in table 4.1.7 (a) revealed that majority earning members were two (45.7%) and one (27.7%). Three earning members comprised 15.3% of the sample, whereas more than three earning members comprise just 11.4% of the sample.

Table 4.1.7 (a) - Earning Members in the household of women in the four BMI categories; (n=387) ; % (n)						
Number of earning members	N (n=90)	PO (n=61)	OW (n=156)	Ob (n=80)	% Total (n=387)	P – value
One (1)	15.9(17)	26.2(28)	41.1(44)	16.8(18)	27.7 (107)	0.001 (S)
Two (2)	23.2(41)	15.8(28)	38.4(68)	22.6(40)	45.7 (177)	
Three (3)	13.6(8)	8.5(5)	47.5(28)	30.5(18)	15.3 (59)	
> Three	54.5 (24)	0	36.4 (16)	9.1 (4)	11.4 (44)	
Parentheses indicate number of subjects. The level of significance for Chi-square was taken as p<0.05); (S) indicates Significant.						

The mean number of earning family members was highest for N and lowest for PO as shown in Table 4.1.7 (b).

Table 4.1.7 (b) - Mean number of earning members in the four BMI categories; (n=387) (mean ± SD with range)					
Mean earning members	N (n=90)	PO (n=61)	OW (n=156)	Ob (n=80)	Total (n=387)
	2.74 ± 1.6 (1-6)	1.62 ± 0.637 (1-3)	2.15 ± 1.04 (1-5)	2.10 ± 0.81 (1-4)	2.19 ± 1.2 (1-6)

The four BMI categories differed significantly (p=0.001) with respect to the number of earning members.

The monthly family income of 91.7% of the sample was more than Rs.50,000/- as depicted in table 4.1.7 (c).

Table 4.1.7 (c) - Monthly family income of women in four BMI categories; (n=387) ; % (n)					
Monthly Income	N (n=90)	PO (n=61)	OW (n=156)	Ob (n=80)	% Total (n=387)
40,000 – 65,000	43.8(12)	0	50.0(16)	6.2(2)	8.3 (32)
>65,000	21.4(76)	17.2(61)	39.4(140)	22.0(78)	91.7 (355)
Parentheses indicate number of subjects.					

4.2 HEALTH PROFILE AND CO-MORBIDITIES

The health profile of the subjects included questions on family history of disease, reproductive and general health including their own perception regarding their weight status. Also, the information relating to weight reducing techniques used by subjects was elucidated. The results have been tabulated in Table 4.2.1 to Table 4.2.9.

4.2.1 Family history of chronic degenerative diseases

Positive family history of disease is an important non-modifiable risk factor for chronic degenerative diseases (NCEP, 1994). In the present study the subjects were asked about the family history of seven non-communicable diseases. The results of which are given in Table 4.2.1.

Table 4.2.1 - Percentage prevalence of disease in family of the women in four BMI categories; (n=387) {% (n)}

Disease	N (n=90)	PO (n=61)	OW (n=156)	Ob (n=80)	% Total (n=387)	P - value
Obesity	0.8 (1)	4.8 (6)	59.5 (75)	34.9 (44)	32.6 (126)	0.001 (S)
Hypertension	15.0 (24)	12.5 (20)	50.0 (80)	22.5 (36)	41.3 (160)	0.001 (S)
Heart Disease (CVD)	13.8 (16)	15.5 (18)	44.0 (51)	26.7 (31)	30.0 (116)	0.018 (S)
Diabetes	17.9 (20)	10.7 (12)	44.6 (50)	26.8 (30)	28.9 (112)	0.041 (S)
Arthritis	17.2 (10)	22.4 (13)	24.1 (14)	36.2 (21)	15.0 (58)	0.002 (S)
Asthma	10.0 (2)	70.0 (14)	20.0 (4)	0	5.2 (20)	0.001 (S)
Any Other	0	0	100 (14)	0	3.6 (14)	0.001 (S)

Parentheses indicate number of subjects.
The level of significance was taken as $p<0.05$; (S) indicates Significant.

Family history of obesity was reported by 33% (n=126) of the subjects, of which 60% (n=75) were in the OW group and 35% (n=44) were in the Ob group. Just one subject (0.8%) in the N group reported family history of obesity and only 4.8% (n=6) of the subjects with a family history of obesity belonged to the PO group. OW and Ob had significant (p=0.001) family history of obesity as compared to PO and N. Thus, indicating that family history of obesity is an important risk factor for developing overweight / obesity.

A total of 160 (41.3%) participants reported a family history of hypertension, of which 50% (n=80) of the participants belonged to OW category, followed by 22.5% (n=36) to the Ob. Only 15% and 12.5% belonging to N and PO category respectively reported family history of hypertension. Again OW and Ob category had significantly higher (p=0.001) family history of hypertension as compared to PO and N.

The 116 (30%) study subjects reported family history of cardio vascular disease (CVD). Data revealed that 44% (n=51) belonged to the OW category and 27% (n=30) to the Ob group. There was a significant difference (p=0.018) between BMI categories with respect to the family history of heart disease, which was higher in OW and Ob than PO and N.

A total of 112 (28.9%) subjects reported family history of diabetes, of which 44.6% (n=50) belonged to the OW category, 26.8% to the Ob, 17.9% to N and 10.7% to PO category. There was a significant difference (p=0.041) between BMI categories with respect to family history of diabetes. CVD, hypertension and T2DM are all co-morbidities associated with obesity. The data on family history of these co-morbidities in the present study indicates that the family history of these diseases is a significant factor affecting weight status of the subjects in the present study.

The data on family history of hyperthyroidism and hypothyroidism was very small to draw a conclusion with respect to its significance. Just 2.3% (n=9) of the total participants reported family history of hyperthyroidism. Out of these 9 subjects, 4 subjects each belonged to the PO and OW category and the remaining one subject belonged to the N category. Like hyperthyroidism, family history of hypothyroidism was reported by just 8 (2.1%) subjects and none of the OW and Ob category subjects reported family history of hypothyroidism. It is possible that the subjects were unaware regarding the family history of hyper and hypothyroidism.

There was a significant difference (p=0.002) between BMI categories with respect to the family history of arthritis. Higher number of subjects from the Ob category (36.2%; n=21) reported family history of arthritis, followed by 24.1% (n=14) from OW, 22.4% (n=13) from PO and 17.2% (n=10) from N category. Thus indicating that prevalence of family history of arthritis is significantly higher (p=0.002) amongst OW and Ob BMI category subjects.

Just 5.2% (n=20) of the total participants reported family history of asthma, of which 70% (n=14) belonged to Po, 20% (n=4) to OW 10.2% (n=2) to N and none to the Ob

BMI category. Although a very small number of subjects reported family history of asthma, but was significantly higher (p=0.001) for PO and OW as compared to N.

Family history of problems like osteoporosis and difficulty in conception by parents were also reported by 14 subjects in the OW category. The study of family history of NCD is important because presence of a positive family history being not modifiable will influence the intensity of risk factor management of the subjects.

More number of subjects in the OW and Ob category as compared to PO and N reported family history of obesity/excess weight, cardiovascular disease, hypertension, type-2 diabetes and arthritis. Family history of asthma was significantly higher for PO category. Therefore, it can be said that the family history of NCD is a significant factor affecting weight status of subjects in the present study.

4.2.2 Weight status of parents of the women in the study group

The present study studied the weight status of parents together with that of the subjects; dividing them into three categories, viz. normal, overweight and underweight.

It was noted that none of the 387 subjects grouped their parents in the underweight category. Table 4.2.2 (a) gives weight status of mother.

4.2.2 (a) Weight status of mother of women in the four BMI categories; n=387; % (n)

Weight Status	N (n=90)	PO (n=61)	OW (n=156)	Ob (n=80)	% Total (n=387)	P – value
Normal	31.5 (80)	17.7 (45)	35.8 (91)	15.0 (38)	65.6 (254)	< 0.001 (S)
Overweight	7.5 (10)	12.0 (16)	48.9 (65)	31.6 (42)	34.4 (133)	
Underweight	0	0	0	0	0	

Parentheses indicate number of subjects.
The level of significance was taken as $p<0.05$; (S) indicates Significant

It was observed that 65.6% (n=254) women reported the weight of their mother as normal, of which 31.5% (n=80) belonged to N, whereas 34.4% (n=133) subjects reported overweight status of their mother of which nearly half (48.9%; n=65) belonged to OW and 31.6% (n=42) to Ob. Thus the percentage women reporting overweight status of mother was significantly higher (p<0.001) for OW and Ob as compared to PO and N. The weight status of father as reported by the subjects has been given in table 4.2.2 (b). It was observed that out of 134 (34.6%) women reporting overweight status of their father, more than half (61.1%; n=88) belonged to OW and 21.5% (n=31) to Ob. Just 11.1% to PO and only 6.2% to N. Like maternal weight status, the overweight status of father was significantly higher (p<0.001) for subjects belonging to OW and Ob as compared to PO and N.

4.2.2 (b) Weight status of father of women in the four BMI categories; n=387; % (n)

Weight Status	N (n=90)	PO (n=61)	OW (n=156)	Ob (n=80)	% Total (n=387)	P – value
Normal	33.3 (81)	18.5 (45)	28.0 (68)	20.2 (49)	62.8 (243)	
Overweight	6.2 (9)	11.1 (16)	61.1 (88)	21.5 (31)	34.6 (134)	< 0.001 (S)
Underweight	0	0	0	0	0	

Parentheses indicate number of subjects.
The level of significance was taken as p<0.05; (S) indicates Significant; (NS) indicates Not Significant

Thus in the present study weight status of parents was a significant factor affecting the weight status of the subjects.

4.2.3 Reproductive health of the women in the four BMI categories

Reproductive health is a condition in which the reproductive process is accomplished in a state of complete physical, mental and social well being and is not merely the absence of disease or disorders of the reproductive process. It also includes the health beyond the child bearing years (Sadana, 2002). In the present study questions related to age of menarche, regularity of menstrual cycle, parity, breast feeding and weight gain after parity were asked. The results have been tabulated in Table 4.2.3.1 to 4.2.3.8.

4.2.3.1 Age of onset of menarche

The mean age of onset of menarche for the subjects belonging to PO (12.72 ± 1.03 y), OW (13.05 ± 0.95 y) and Ob (13.38 ± 1.04 y) category was lower than that of the subjects belonging to N (13.5 ± 0.58 y) category as depicted in Table 4.2.3.1. The data revealed that the mean age of menarche was significantly lower ($p<0.001$) for PO, OW and Ob as compared to N. Thus in the present study age of onset of menarche was a significant factor affecting weight status of the subjects.

Table 4.2.3.1 Mean age of onset of menarche of the women in the four BMI categories; (n=387) (mean ± SD with range)

	N (n=90)	PO (n=61)	OW (n=156)	Ob (n=80)	Total (n=387)	P – value
Mean age of onset of Menarche (Years)	13.5 ± 0.58[a] (13-15)	12.72 ± 1.03[b] (11-14)	13.05 ± 0.96[c] (11-15)	13.38 ± 1.05[d] (12-15)	13.17 ± 0.953 (11-15)	<0.001 (S)

The level of significance for ANOVA was taken as $p<0.05$; (S) indicates Significant;
Age of menarche; (ANOVA)
[a] – N > PO, OW ; [b] – PO < N, OW, Ob ; [c] – OW < N, Ob ; [d] – Ob < N, Ob > PO, OW

4.2.3.2 Regularity of menstrual cycle

When the subjects were enquired about the regularity of menstrual cycle, it was observed that out of 387 women, 90.7% (n=351) reported regular menstruation. In this group all the 90 women (25.6%) belonging to N category were having regular menstrual cycle, but 12 women each (33.3%) belonging to PO, OW and Ob category reported having irregular menstrual cycle. The results have been tabulated in Table 4.2.3.2.

Table 4.2.3.2 - Regularity of menstrual cycle of the women in the four BMI categories; n=387; % (n)

Menstrual Cycle	N (n=90)	PO (n=61)	OW (n=156)	Ob (n=80)	% Total (n=387)	P – value
Regular	25.6 (90)	14.0 (49)	41.0 (144)	19.4 (68)	90.7 (351)	0.022 (S)
Irregular	0	33.3 (12)	33.3 (12)	33.3 (12)	9.3 (36)	

Parentheses indicate number of subjects.
The level of significance was taken as $p<0.05$; (S) indicates significant.

Regularity in menstrual cycle was significantly higher (p=0.022) for the N BMI category as compared to the other overweight categories. Thus, reflecting that any imbalance or irregularity in menstruation effects weight status. Regular menstruation was a significant factor for weight status of subjects in the present study.

4.2.3.3 Age of marriage of the study subjects

The mean of marriage of the subjects has been given in table 4.2.3.3. Age of marriage was a significant factor (p=0.001) for the subjects in four BMI categories. It was observed that the mean age of marriage was lowest for women belonging to Ob category at 23.8 years, followed by OW at 24.2 years. It was 24.7 years and 25.6 years for N and PO category respectively. Thus women belonging to Ob and OW category got married at a younger age than women in N and PO categories.

Table 4.2.3.3 - Mean age of marriage of the women in the four BMI categories; (n=387) (mean ± SD with range)

	N (n=90)	PO (n=61)	OW (n=156)	Ob (n=80)	Total (n=387)	P – value
Mean age of Marriage	24.78 $\pm$ 2.60^{a} (20-30)	25.62 $\pm$ 2.49^{b} (19-39)	24.21 $\pm$ 2.73^{c} (20-31)	23.86 $\pm$ 3.00^{d} (18-29)	24.49 $\pm$ 2.77 18-39)	0.001 (S)

The level of significance for ANOVA was taken as p<0.05; (S) indicates Significant.
Age of marriage; (ANOVA)
^{a}– N > Ob ; ^{b}– PO > OW, Ob ; ^{c}– OW < PO ; ^{d}– Ob < N, PO

4.2.3.4 Age at parity

Age at parity also came out as a significant factor (p<0.001) for weight status of subjects in the present study as shown in table 4.2.3.4. As reported earlier, that the mean age of marriage for the subjects in the obese group was the lowest amongst the four BMI categories. So was their mean age at parity. The mean age of women in the study sample at the time of first parity was 26.09 $\pm$ 3.219 years. For women in the Ob, OW, N and Po category, it was 25.19 $\pm$ 3.073, 25.89 $\pm$ 2.793, 26.31 $\pm$ 4.169 and 27.5 $\pm$ 2.241 years respectively. Also, the mean age of women belonging to Ob and OW category was significantly lower (p<0.001) than that of N and PO category at the time of last parity. The mean age of women at the time of last parity in Ob, OW, N and Po

BMI categories was 26.65 $\pm$ 6.156, 28.06 $\pm$ 1.537, 29.56 $\pm$ 2.822 and 30.28 $\pm$ 1.88 years respectively. Since the women in the obese group not only got married at a younger age, but also became mothers at a younger age than women in other BMI categories. The younger age at parity for OW and Ob was a significant factor ($p<0.001$) affecting weight status of the women in the study.

Table 4.2.3.4 - Mean age of women in the four BMI categories at parity; (n=387) (mean ± SD with range)

Mean age at parity	N (n=90)	PO (n=61)	OW (n=156)	Ob (n=80)	Total (n=387)	P – value
First parity	26.3 $\pm$ 4.17 [a] (22-33)	27.5 $\pm$ 2.24 [b] (23-40)	25.89 $\pm$ 2.79 [c] (21-32)	25.19 $\pm$ 3.07 [d] (20-30)	26.09 $\pm$ 3.22 (20-40)	<0.001 (S)
Last parity	29.56 $\pm$ 2.82 [a-1] (25-34)	30.28 $\pm$ 1.89 [b-1] (26-33)	28.06 $\pm$ 1.54 [c-1] (24-31)	26.65 $\pm$ 6.16 [d-1] (24-35)	28.25 $\pm$ 4.03 (24-35)	<0.001 (S)

The level of significance for ANOVA was taken as $p<0.05$; (S) indicates Significant.
Age at first parity; (ANOVA)
[a] – N < PO, N > Ob ; [b] – PO > N, OW, Ob ; [c] – OW < PO ; [d] – Ob < N, PO
Age at second parity; (ANOVA)
[a-1] – N > OW, Ob ; [b-1] – PO > OW, Ob ; [C-1] – OW < N, PO, OW > Ob ; [d-1] – Ob < N, PO, OW

4.2.3.5 Occurrence of miscarriage in the study group

A total of 30.2% (117) women of the study sample reported having miscarriage. The data has been given in tables 4.2.3.5 (a) and (b). The mean number of miscarriages reported by 117 women was 1.5 $\pm$ 0.639. The four BMI categories did not differ significantly ($p=0.752$) with respect to the mean number of miscarriages. However, the frequency of miscarriage was significantly more ($p=0.005$) for the women belonging to OW and Ob category as compared to PO and N category. Out of the 117 women reporting miscarriage 40.2% (n=47) belonged to OW and 30.8% (n=36) belonged to Ob category. It was also observed that 30.1% of the OW and 45.0% of Ob women experienced miscarriage as compared to just 24.6% of PO and only 21.1% of N. Thus miscarriage was a significant outcome of overweight and obese status of the subjects in the study.

Table 4.2.3.5 (a) Percentage women in the study group reporting miscarriage; (n=387) {% (n)}						
% Women experiencing miscarriage	N (n=90)	PO (n=61)	OW (n=156)	Ob (n=80)	% Total (n=387)`	P – value
% of total sample	16.2 (19)	12.8 (15)	40.2 (47)	30.8 (36)	30.2 (117)	0.005 (S)
% within group	21.1 (19)	24.6 (15)	30.1 (47)	45.0 (36)		
Parentheses indicate number of subjects. The level of significance for Chi-square was taken as $p<0.05$; (S) indicates Significant.						

Table 4.2.3.5 (b) Mean number of miscarriages in the four BMI categories; (n=117) (mean ± SD with range)						
Number of miscarriages	N (n=19)	PO (n=15)	OW (n=47)	Ob (n=36)	Total (n=117)	P – value
	1.53 ± 0.697 (1-2)	1.40 ± 0.507 (1-2)	1.46 ± 0.504 (1-2)	1.58 ± 0.806 (1-2)	1.5 ± 0.639 (1-2)	0.752 (NS)
The level of significance for ANOVA was taken as $p<0.05$; (NS) indicates Not Significant						

4.2.3.6 Use of oral contraceptives

Use of oral contraceptives was a significant factor (p=0.004) for weight gain as shown in table 4.2.3.6 (a). Although a small percentage of women in study sample, i.e 20.9% (n=81) reported the use of oral contraceptives as a means of birth control but 55.6% of this group belonged to OW category. Remaining 17.3%, 14.8% and 12.3% belonged to Ob, PO and N categories respectively.

Likewise, when self reported side effects associated with the use of oral contraceptives were studied and depicted in table 4.2.3.6 (c), The data revealed that out of the 81 women reporting weight gain after consumption of oral contraceptives, 62.7% (n=42) belonged to OW category, and 20.8% (n=14) belonged to the Ob. Weight gain as a side effect was also reported by 11.9% and 4.5% women belonging to PO and N categories.

Weight gain as a side effect of use of consumption of oral contraceptives was as a significant factor (p=0.001) affecting the weight status of the subjects in the study. The mean duration of intake of oral contraceptives was 14.6 ± 10.34 months for the study sample. The four BMI categories did not differ significantly (p=0.567) with respect to the duration of consumption of oral contraceptives. In the present study, duration of intake of oral contraceptives did not come out as a significant factor affecting weight status of the subjects. The data has been given in table 4.2.3.6 (b).

Table 4.2.3.6 (a) Percentage women using oral contraceptives in the four BMI categories; (n=387) {% (n)}

% Women using oral contraceptives	N (n=90)	PO (n=61)	OW (n=156)	Ob (n=80)	% Total (n=387)	P – value
% of total sample	12.3 (10)	14.8 (12)	55.6 (45)	17.3 (14)	20.9 (81)	0.004 (S)
% within group	11.1 (10)	21.4 (12)	28.9 8 (45)	17.5 (14)		

The level of significance for Chi-square was taken as $p<0.05$; (S) indicates Significant.

Table 4.2.3.6 (b) Mean duration of intake of oral contraceptives by the women in the four BMI categories; (n=81) (mean ± SD with range)

	N (n=10)	PO (n=12)	OW (n=45)	Ob (n=14)	Total (n=81)	P – value
Duration of intake of oral contraceptive (months)	15.25 ± 15.17 (6-24)	14.92 ± 10.31 (5-36)	15.43 ± 8.85 (6-30)	11.13 ± 10.69 (3-36)	14.6 ± 10.34 (3-36)	0.567 (NS)

The level of significance for ANOVA was taken as $p<0.05$; (NS) indicates Not Significant

Table 4.2.3.6 (c) Side effects of oral contraceptives among the women in the four BMI categories; n=81; % (n)

Side effects	N (n=10)	PO (n=12)	OW (n=45)	Ob (n=14)	% Total (n=81)	P –value
Weight Gain	4.5 (3)	11.9 (8)	62.7 (42)	20.8 (14)	82.7 (67)	0.001 (S)
Weight Loss	66.7 (2)	0	0	0	2.5 (2)	
No side effects	41.7 (5)	33.3 (4)	25.0 (3)	0	14.8 (12)	

The level of significance for Chi-square was taken as $p<0.05$; (S) indicates Significant.

4.2.3.7 Breast feeding

Out of the 387 study subjects, 97.7% (n=378) reported that they breast fed their infants. The within group analysis as shown in table 4.2.3.7 revealed that all women in N and PO category were able to breast feed as compared to 98.1% of OW and 92.5% of Ob. The six Ob and three OW women, who were unable to breast feed their infants reported that they were put on strong antibiotics and were recommended not to breastfeed their child. Thus the inability to breast feed was a significant outcome (p=0.004) of overweight and obese status of the subjects in the present study. Significant number of women in OW and Ob category were unable to breastfeed their children as compared to N and PO.

Table 4.2.3.7 Percentage women in the four BMI categories who breast fed their children; n=387; % (n)

Women breast feeding	N (n=90)	PO (n=61)	OW (n=156)	Ob (n=80)	% Total (n=387)	P – value
% in the study sample	23.8 (90)	16.1 (61)	40.5 (153)	19.6 (74)	97.7 (378)	0.004 (S)
% within group	100.0 (90)	100.0 (61)	98.1 (153)	92.5 (74)		

The level of significance for Chi-square was taken as p<0.05; (S) indicates significant.

4.2.3.8 Post partum weight gain in the study group

Out of the 387 women, 81.7% (n=316) women reported having gained weight after child birth as shown in Table 4.2.3.8 (a), it was noted that all the Ob subjects and 87.8% of the OW women reported post partum weight gain as compared to 67.2% and 64.4% of PO and N respectively. Significantly, higher number of women (p<0.001) belonging to OW and Ob reported post partum weight gain as compared to women in N and PO.

Table 4.2.3.8 (a) Percentage women reporting post partum weight gain in the four BMI categories; n=387; % (n)

Post Partum Weight Gain	N (n=90)	PO (n=61)	OW (n=156)	Ob (n=80)	% Total (n=387)	P – value
% in the study sample	18.4 (58)	13.0 (41)	43.4 (137)	25.3 (80)	81.6 (316)	<0.001 (S)
% within group	64.4 (58)	67.2 (41)	87.8 (137)	100.0 (80)		

The level of significance for Chi-square was taken as p<0.05; (S) indicates significant.

Similarly, when the mean post partum weight gain amongst the four categories was evaluated, it was observed that mean weight gain after first parity was highest for women belonging to Ob, followed by OW as given in Table 4.2.3.8 (b). However, the mean weight gain after 2nd parity was highest for Ob but the 2nd highest gain was for PO, although, closely followed by OW. The mean weight gain after each parity was significantly higher ($p<0.001$; $p=0.001$) for the subjects belonging to PO, OW and Ob as compared to N. From the data, it can be commented that a post partum weight gain of 3-4 kg keeps the women in the normal weight category, whereas weight gain beyond this limit as observed from Table 4.2.3.8 (b) leads to overweight/obese status.

Table 4.2.3.8 (b) Mean weight gain after first and second parity in four BMI categories; (n=138) (mean ± SD with range)

Weight Gain after parity (Kg)	N (n=28)	PO (n=19)	OW (n=57)	Ob (n=34)	Total (n=138)	P – value
First Parity	4.82 ± 2.6 (2-5)	4.81 ± 0.4 (4-10)	6.88 ± 3.78 (1-15)	11.76 ± 3.97 (5-20)	7.5 ± 4.3 (1-20)	<0.001(S)
Second Parity	3.3 ± 1.3 (2-5)	8.0 ± 0.00 (8-8)	7.31 ± 2.62 (2-10)	10.57 ± 2.2 (6-16)	7.65 ± 3.24 (2-16)	0.001 (S)

The level of significance for ANOVA was taken as $p<0.05$; (S) indicates significant.

4.2.4 Health monitoring

When the 387 women were inquired about the various health parameters being monitored by them, it revealed that 94.3% (n=365) women were just monitoring their blood pressure at home or at the neighborhood clinic. Amongst these, 40.5% (n=148) belonged to OW, 21.9% (n=80) to Ob, 20.8% (n=76) to N and 16.7% (n=61) to PO. There was a significant difference ($p<0.001$) between the four BMI categories with respect to health monitoring. The results have been tabulated in table 4.2.4. All the women belonging to PO and Ob were monitoring their health as compared to 84.4% of N and 94.9% of OW. The present study revealed that health monitoring was a significant factor and generally the subjects were health conscious.

Table 4.2.4 Percentage women monitoring health in four BMI categories; n=387; % (n)						
Health Monitoring	N (n=90)	PO (n=61)	OW (n=156)	Ob (n=80)	% Total (n=387)	P – value
% in the study sample	20.8 (76)	16.7 (61)	40.5 (148)	21.9 (80)	94.3 (365)	<0.001 (S)
% within group	84.4 (76)	100.0 (61)	94.9 (148)	100.0 (80)		
The level of significance for Chi-square was taken as p<0.05; (S) indicates significant.						

4.2.5 Co-morbidities

Health status of the subjects was analysed from the secondary data available with the subjects. The secondary data included blood-pressure reports and blood test reports, if performed in last six months. Tables 4.2.5 (a), (b) and (c) gives the health status of the subjects with respect to blood pressure, blood glucose and blood cholesterol.

As observed from table 4.2.5 (a), out of the 365 women, who were monitoring their blood pressure 30.1% (n=110) were pre-hypertensive i.e. systolic blood pressure (SBP) value between 120-139 mmHg or diastolic blood pressure (DBP) value between 80-89 mmHg. (Chobanian et al, 2003). The cutoff values for blood pressure is given in **Annexure – 8.** Amongst these 55.5% (n=61) belonged to Ob and 44.5% (n=49) belonged to OW. None belonged to N and PO categories. Also, 3 women belonging to Ob category were in stage I hypertension i.e. SBP value between 140-159 mmHg. or DBP value between 90-94 mmHg. There was a significant difference (p<0.001) amongst the four BMI categories with respect to hypertension. However, withing group data revealed that significantly higher (p<0.001) women in N (84.4%) had blood pressure value within normal range as compared to just 20.0% of Ob.

Table 4.2.5 (b) depicts the fasting blood glucose data. Out of the 343 women who gave the secondary data for fasting blood glucose, 12 (3.5%) women had impaired fasting glucose i.e. fasting plasma glucose (FPG) between 100-125 mg/dl (ADA, 2003). Cutoff values for plasma blood glucose is given in **Annexure – 9**. Amongst these, 7 women (4.5%) were in OW and 5 women (6.3%) were in Ob category. But none belonged to N and PO category. There was a significant difference (p=0.037) amongst the four BMI categories with respect to fasting blood glucose values.

Table 4.2.5 (a) Co-morbidity (Blood Pressure) of women in the four BMI categories; n=365; % (n)

Blood Pressure		N (n=76)	PO (n=61)	OW (n=148)	Ob (n=80)	% Total (n=365)	P – value
Within Normal Range (<120/<80mm Hg)	% in sample	30.3 (76)	24.2 (61)	39.4 (99)	6.1 (16)	69.04 (252)	<0.001 (S)
	% within group	84.4 (76)	100 (61)	63.5 (99)	20.0 (16)		
Pre-Hypertension (120-139/80-89 mmHg)	% in sample	0	0	44.5 (49)	55.5 (61)	30.14 (110)	
	% within group	0	0	31.4 (49)	76.3 (61)		
Hypertension (140-159/90-94 mmHg)	% in sample	0	0	0	100.0 (3)	0.84 (3)	
	% within group	0	0	0	3.8 (3)		

The level of significance for Chi-square was taken as p<0.05; (S) indicates significant.

Table 4.2.5 (b) Co-morbidity (Blood Glucose) of women in the four BMI categories; n=343; % (n)

Blood Glucose		N (n=75)	PO (n=61)	OW (n=133)	Ob (n=74)	% Total (n=343)	P – value
Normal (70-100) {mg./dl.}	% in sample	22.7 (75)	18.4 (61)	38.1 (126)	20.8 (69)	96.5 (331)	0.037 (S)
	% within group	83.3 (75)	100 (61)	80.0 (126)	86.3 (69)		
Impaired FPG > 100 {mg./dl.}	% in sample	0	0	58.3 (7)	41.7 (5)	3.5 (12)	
	% within group	0	0	4.5 (7)	6.3 (5)		

The level of significance for Chi-square was taken as p<0.05; (S) indicates significant.

Similarly, secondary data of total blood cholesterol, as shown in table 4.2.5 (c), was obtained from 271 women, amongst which 56.8% (n=154) women were having border line high cholesterol i.e. total blood cholesterol value between 200-239 mg/dl (NCEP, 2004). The cutoff values for blood cholesterol is given in **Annexure – 10**. Surprisingly, amongst these 31.8% (n=49) belonged to PO, 27.9% (n=43) belonged to OW, 22.1% (n=34) to N and 18.2% (n=28) to Ob category. Thus indicating that women belonging to PO and N category are also at increased risk of developing CVD, though apparently healthy. However, none of the women belonging to N and PO category were hyper-cholestromic, but 14 women 77.8% belonging to OW and 4 women 22.2% belonging to Ob category had their blood cholesterol values ≥ 240 mg/dl. There was a significance difference (p=0.001) between the four BMI categories with respect to the occurrence of high blood cholesterol. Greater number of women in OW and Ob BMI category had their blood cholesterol value higher than the desirable value of < 200 mg/dl.

Obesity related co-morbidities like hypertension, impaired blood glucose and high cholesterol were significantly higher for Ob and OW in the study.

Table 4.2.5 (c) Co-morbidity (Blood Cholesterol) of women in the four BMI categories; n=271; % (n)

Blood Cholesterol		N (n=57)	PO (n=61)	OW (n=111)	Ob (n=42)	% Total (n=271)	P – value
Normal (< 200mg/dl)	% in sample	23.2 (23)	12.1 (12)	54.5 (54)	10.1 (10)	36.5 (99)	0.001 (S)
	% within group	25.6 (23)	19.7 (12)	34.6 (54)	12.5 (10)		
At Risk (200-239 mg/dl)	% in sample	22.1 (34)	31.8 (49)	27.9 (43)	18.2 (28)	56.8 (154)	
	% within group	37.8 (34)	80.3 (49)	27.6 (43)	35.0 (28)		
High Cholesterol (≥ 240 mg/dl)	% in sample	0	0	77.8 (14)	22.2 (4)	6.7 (18)	
	% within group	0	0	9.0 (14)	5.0 (4)		

The level of significance for Chi-square was taken as p<0.05; (S) indicates significant.

4.2.6 Prescribed treatment for obesity and associated co-morbidities

Table 4.2.6 gives the data on type of treatment prescribed for obesity and associated co-morbidities. It was observed that 74.5% (n=120) of the subjects were prescribed dietary modifications as treatment to deal with obesity related co-morbidities. Also, 64.0% (n=103) of the subjects were prescribed exercise. Specific drug therapy was prescribed to 42.2% (n=68) subjects to manage blood pressure, high cholesterol and hypothyroidism. Vitamin and mineral supplementation was prescribed to just 18 (11.2%) subjects. The data revealed that morbidity was higher in OW and Ob categories.

Table 4.2.6 Percentage women in the four BMI categories who were prescribed treatment for obesity and co morbidities; n=161; % (n)

Type of Treatment	N (n=8)	PO (n=14)	OW (n=92)	Ob (n=47)	% Total (n=161)	P – value
Drug	4.4 (3)	13.2 (9)	57.4 (39)	25.0 (17)	42.2 (68)*	0.311 (NS)
Exercise	1.0 (1)	0	66.0 (68)	33.0 (34)	64.0 (103)*	0.001 (S)
Diet Modification	4.2 (5)	3.3 (4)	64.2 (77)	28.3 (34)	74.5 (120)*	0.001 (S)
Vitamin and Mineral Supplementation	5.6 (1)	16.7 (3)	72.2 (13)	5.6 (1)	11.2 (18)*	0.103 (NS)

*(161 subjects were using more than one type of treatment)

Parentheses indicate number of subjects. The level of significance for Chi-square was taken as $p<0.05$; (S) indicates significant; (NS) indicates not significant

4.2.7 Self perception of weight status

Body image has a significant impact on the weight managing behaviour of women Schwartz and Brownell (2004). In the present study, subjects were asked to group themselves as normal weight, overweight or underweight at present and at pre-marriage time. The results of which have been given in Tables 4.2.7 (a) and (b). It was observed that 29.7% perceived themselves as normal and 70.3% perceived themselves as overweight. Nobody perceived as underweight, but in pre-marriage weight perception, 10.6% perceived themselves as underweight. Also, 73.9% claimed themselves to be normal and only 15.5% claimed to be overweight. Those who were overweight and obese before marriage, all have same BMI categories now.

Comparison of self perception of overweight amongst the women classified as N, PO, OW and Ob revealed that significantly higher ($p<0.001$) number of women belonging to OW (55.1%; n=150) and Ob (28.7%; n=78) BMI category correctly perceived themselves as overweight. However, 12.9% (n=35) women belonging to PO and 3.3% (n=9) belonging to N, incorrectly perceived themselves as overweight.

Table 4.2.7 (a) Self perceived weight status of women in the four BMI categories at present; n=387; % (n)

Perceived Weight Status at present		N (n=90)	PO (n=61)	OW (n=156)	Ob (n=80)	% Total (n=387)	P-value
Underweight	% in sample	0	0	0	0	0	<0.001 (S)
	% within group	0	0	0	0		
Normal	% in sample	70.4 (81)	22.6 (26)	5.2 (6)	1.7 (2)	29.7 (115)	
	% within group	90.0 (81)	42.6 (26)	3.8 (6)	2.5 (2)		
Overweight	% in sample	3.3 (9)	12.9 (35)	55.1 (150)	28.7 (78)	70.3 (272)	
	% within group	10.0 (9)	57.4 (35)	96.2 (150)	97.5 (78)		

The level of significance for Chi-square was taken as $p<0.05$; (S) indicates significant.

Table 4.2.7 (b) Pre marriage self perceived weight status of women in four BMI categories; n=387; % (n)

Perceived Pre marriage weight status		N (n=90)	PO (n=61)	OW (n=156)	Ob (n=80)	% Total (n=387)	P-value
Underweight	% in sample	56.1 (23)	12.2 (5)	31.7 (13)	0	10.6 (41)	<0.001 (S)
	% within group	25.6 (23)	8.2 (5)	8.3 (13)	0		
Normal	% in sample	23.4 (61)	19.6 (56)	35.0 (100)	22.0 (63)	73.9 (286)	
	% within group	67.8 (61)	91.8 (56)	64.1 (100)	78.6 (63)		
Overweight	% in sample	0	0	71.7 (43)	28.3 (17)	15.5 (60)	
	% within group	0	0	27.6 (43)	21.3 (17)		

The level of significance for Chi-square was taken as $p<0.05$; (S) indicates significant.

4.2.8 Change in weight status in last one year

Weight status of the subjects was also evaluated in terms of weight lost or gained in last one year. The self reported mean weight gain or loss as reported by 387 women has been given in table 4.2.8. It revealed that the mean weight gain was significantly higher (p<0.001) for Ob (7.6 Kg) and OW (4.8 Kg) as compared to PO (3.19 Kg) and N (3.16 Kg). It is possible that N and PO category might not have gained this amount of weight in just one year, but gradually over a period of time. In contrast OW and Ob reported weight gain of 4.88 Kg and 7.68 Kg respectively. This reflects that a weight gain of 5.7 Kg in one year can lead to overweight and obese status, whereas 3 Kg weight gain/loss per annum ensures normal weight.

In the present study, higher weight gain (5-7 Kg) per annum and lower weight loss (2-3 Kg) per annum was a significant factor (p<0.001) affecting the weight status of the subjects.

Table 4.2.8 Mean weight gained and lost in kilograms in last one year by women in four BMI categories; (n=224) (mean ± SD with range)

Mean weight gained/lost	N (n=50)	PO (n=31)	OW (n=96)	Ob (n=47)	Total (n=224)	P-value
Weight Lost (Kg)	3.27 ± 1.37 (1-5) (n=31)	2.93 ± 1.21 (2-5) (n=16)	3.70 ± 1.25 (2-5) (n=38)	2.2 ± 0.45 (2-3) (n=9)	3.16 ± 1.29 (1-5) (n=94)	0.158 (NS)
Weight Gain (Kg)	3.16 ± 1.07 (2-5) (n=19)	3.19 ± 1.36 (2-5) (n=15)	4.88 ± 1.72 (1-10) (n=58)	7.68 ± 4.55 (3-20) (n=38)	5.13 ± 3.22 (1-20) (n=130)	<0.001 (S)

The level of significance for ANOVA was taken as p<0.05;
(S) indicates significant; (NS) indicates not significant

4.2.9 Adoption of weight reducing techniques

More than half i.e 52.5% (n=203) women reported adopting various weight reducing techniques as shown in Table 4.2.9 (a). Among these, 58.6% (n=119) women belonged to OW, 22.7% (n=46) to Ob and 9.4% (n=19) each to N and PO category. The within group analysis of BMI categories with respect to weight reduction also revealed the similar trend. As high as 76.2% of OW and 57.5% of Ob women were resorting to various weight reducing techniques as compared to just 21.1% and 31.2% of N and PO respectively. The practice of adopting weight reducing techniques was significantly higher ($p<0.001$) for OW and Ob. Also, Table 4.2.9 (b) depicts the data on preference of subjects for various weight reducing techniques in the four BMI categories. The data revealed that the most preferred technique was dietary modification (26.1%) followed by going to gymnasium (18.1%).

Table 4.2.9 (a) Percentage women using weight reducing techniques in four BMI categories; n=387; % (n)

%Women using weight reducing techniques	N (n=90)	PO (n=61)	OW (n=156)	Ob (n=80)	%Total (n=387)	P-value
% in the sample	9.4 (19)	9.4 (19)	58.6 (119)	22.7 (46)	52.5 (203)	<0.001 (S)
% within group	21.1(19)	31.2(19)	76.2(119)	57.5(46)		

The level of significance for Chi-square was taken as $p<0.05$; (S) indicates significant.

Table 4.2.9 (b) Preference for various weight reducing techniques by the women in the four BMI categories; n=387; % (n)

Weight reducing techniques	N (n=90)	PO (n=61)	OW (n=156)	Ob (n=80)	% Total (n=387)	P-value
Pills and Powders	0	0	85.0 (17)	15.0 (3)	5.2 (20)	<0.001 (S)
Gels and Creams	0	0	0	0	0	-
Belt	0	0	0	0	0	-
Health Walker	0	0	25.0 (3)	75.0 (9)	3.1 (12)	<0.001 (S)
Treadmill	0	0	87.2 (34)	12.8 (5)	10.1 (39)	<0.001 (S)
Exercise	13.3 (8)	8.3 (5)	53.3 (32)	25.0 (15)	15.5 (60)	0.028 (S)
Modified Diet	9.9 (10)	5.0 (5)	60.4 (61)	24.8 (25)	26.1 (101)	<0.001 (S)
Gymnasium	5.7 (4)	28.6 (20)	60.0 (42)	5.7 (4)	18.1 (70)	<0.001 (S)
Health Clinic	0	0	54,5 (6)	45.5 (5)	2.8 (11)	0.039 (S)
Any Other	0	0	100.0 (14)	0	3.6 (14)	<0.001 (S)

The level of significance for Chi-square was taken as $p<0.05$; (S) indicates significant.

4.3 DIETARY HISTORY

Diet history gives an insight into the usual food pattern and food habits of the study population. It is essential to study the food pattern and food preferences of the people because diet plays a key role as a risk factor for chronic diseases (WHO, 2003).

In the present study, the dietary history of the study sample was analysed for food preferences during pregnancy and lactation; because parity was an essential inclusion criteria. Out of the 387 women, 14.2% (n=55) had their last parity within last one year. Among these the highest number belonged to N (40.0%; n=22) as shown in table 4.3.

Table 4.3 Percentage women within one year of parity in the four BMI categories; n=387; % (n)

	N (n=90)	PO (n=61)	OW (n=156)	Ob (n=80)	% Total (n=387)	P – value
Last parity within last 1 Year	40.0 (22)	9.1 (5)	32.7 (18)	18.2 (10)	14.2 (55)	0.001 (S)

Parentheses indicate number of subjects; (S) indicates significant.
The level of significance for Chi-square test was taken as $p<0.05$.

4.3.1 Dietary pattern during pregnancy

Diet plays an important role for weight gain during pregnancy but also affect the post pregnancy weight status of the woman. Therefore, the dietary behaviour of women related to types of food included/excluded and reasons for the same during pregnancy and lactation have been analysed in tables 4.3.1.1 to 4.3.1.3.

4.3.1.1 Special food consumed during pregnancy

Table 4.3.1.1 gives the list of special foods consumed by women in the study sample. The highest preference (52.0%; n=200) was seen for protein rich food, followed by preference for fruits and salads (41.1%; n=159). The consumption of protein rich foods was significantly higher ($p<0.001$) for women belonging to OW (37.5%; n=75) and Ob (29.5%; n=59) as compared to N (24.0%; n=48) and PO (9.0%; n=18).

Whereas, the consumption for fruits and salads during pregnancy was significantly higher ($p<0.001$) for OW (36.5%; n=58) and N (28.3%; n=45) as compared to Ob. Also 19.1% (n=74) women in the study sample reported consuming *ghee* during the last trimester.

Table 4.3.1.1 - Special foods consumed by women in the 4 BMI categories during pregnancy; n=387; % (n)

Food		N (n=90)	PO (n=61)	OW (n=156)	Ob (n=80)	% Total (n=387)	P – value
No Special Food	% in sample	13.6 (11)	28.4 (23)	42.0 (34)	16.0 (13)	20.9 (81)	<0.001 (S)
	% within group	12.2 (11)	37.3 (23)	21.8 (34)	16.3 (13)		
Protein Rich Food	% in sample	24.0 (48)	9.0 (18)	37.5 (75)	29.5 (59)	51.8 (200)	<0.001 (S)
	% within group	53.3 (48)	29.5 (18)	48.1 (75)	73.8 (59)		
Fruits/Juice/ Salads	% in sample	28.3 (45)	12.6 (20)	36.5 (58)	22.6 (36)	41.1 (159)	<0.001 (S)
	% within group	50.0 (45)	32.8 (20)	37.2 (58)	45.0 (36)		
Sugar Rich Foods	% in sample	22.7 (5)	0	40.9 (9)	36.4 (8)	5.7 (22)	<0.001 (S)
	% within group	5.6 (5)	0	5.8 (9)	10.0 (8)		
Ghee in last Trimester	% in sample	0	13.5 (10)	54.1 (40)	32.4 (24)	19.1 (74)	<0.001 (S)
	% within group	0	16.4 (10)	25.6 (40)	30.0 (24)		

Parentheses indicate number of subjects; (S) indicates significant.
The level of significance for Chi-square test was taken as $p<0.05$.

Among these, the highest belonged to OW (54.1%; n=40) followed by Ob and PO but none belonged to N. However, within group analysis revealed that significantly higher ($p<0.001$) percentage of Ob women consumed protein rich foods, whereas the consumption of fruits and salads was highest for N (50%). Even the intake of sugar rich food products (10%) and *ghee* (25.6) during pregnancy was highest among Ob women when analysed within group.

Thus the consumption of special foods like eggs, milk, ghee etc has a significant effect on the weight status of the subjects in the present study.

Higher percentage of women belonging to OW and Ob category consumed energy dense foods as compared to the women belonging to N and PO category.

4.3.1.2 Reasons for consuming special foods during pregnancy

The reasons for consuming special foods during pregnancy have been given in table 4.3.1.2. It was observed that out of the 306 women who consumed special foods during pregnancy, almost 62% gave the reason of good health for self and for the growing foetus in the womb. In this group significantly higher ($p<0.001$) number of women belonged to N (36.5%; n=69) as compared to PO, OW and Ob. On the other hand, significantly higher ($p<0.001$) number of women belonging to OW (41.3%; n=33) and Ob (38.8%; n=31) reported consuming special foods on advice of elders as compared to N.

Table 4.3.1.2 - Reasons for consuming special foods during pregnancy by women in the 4 BMI categories; n=306; % (n)

Reasons	N (n=79)	PO (n=38)	OW (n=122)	Ob (n=67)	% Total (n=306)	P – value
Healthy	36.5 (69)	20.1 (38)	27.0 (51)	16.4 (31)	61.8 (189)	<0.001 (S)
On Elder's Advice	20.0 (16)	0	41.3 (33)	38.8 (31)	26.1 (80)	<0.001 (S)
Any Other	67.6 (25)	24.3 (9)	8.1 (3)	0	12.1 (37)	<0.001 (S)

Parentheses indicate number of subjects; (S) indicates significant.
The level of significance for Chi-square test was taken as $p<0.05$.

Also, 12.1% (n=37) women gave reasons like developed liking, doctor's advice for consuming these foods. In this group significantly higher ($p<0.001$) number of women belonged to N as compared to OW and Ob.

4.3.1.3 Foods avoided during pregnancy

Women avoided various kinds of food during pregnancy, which were broadly classified into four categories, namely (i) beverages like tea, coffee, carbonated drinks; (ii) strong smelling foods like onion, garlic, mustard oil, etc; (iii) outside food especially Chinese food and fried food like samosa, pakora etc.; (iv) food fads like avoiding papaya, and food considered hot and can lead to abortion like groundnuts, ajwain etc. The results have been tabulated in table 4.3.1.3. More than half i.e. 61.3% (n=237) of the women did not avoid any kind of foods. Significantly higher (p<0.001) number of women belonged to OW as compared to N, Ob and PO in all the criteria studied.

Table 4.3.1.3 - Foods avoided during pregnancy by the women in the four BMI categories; n=387; % (n)

Food	N (n=90)	PO (n=61)	OW (n=156)	Ob (n=80)	% Total (n=387)	P – value
Nothing Avoided	22.4 (53)	18.6 (44)	39.2 (93)	19.8 (47)	61.3 (237)	<0.001(S)
Beverages	50.0 (19)	0	31.6 (12)	18.4 (7)	9.8 (38)	<0.001(S)
Strong Smelling Foods	15.8 (6)	15.8 (6)	52.6 (20)	15.8 (6)	9.8 (38)	<0.001(S)
Outside Food	18.6 (8)	9.3 (4)	37.2 (16)	34.9 (15)	11.1 (43)	<0.001(S)
Food Fads	12.9 (4)	22.6 (7)	48.4 (15)	16.1 (5)	8.0 (31)	<0.001(S)

Parentheses indicate number of subjects; (S) indicates significant.
The level of significance for Chi-square test was taken as p<0.05.

4.3.2. Dietary pattern during lactation

In India, there is a tradition to feed the mother with energy dense food products like ghee, panjiri, etc., during lactation so that the mother not only gets energy from these products but these products are known to be galactogogues. Apart from this, foods influence the weight status of the mother. Therefore, food preferences of the mother during lactation were studied.

4.3.2.1 Special foods consumed during lactation

Special foods consumed during lactation by the women in the four BMI categories have been given in table 4.3.2.1. It was observed that 76.5% (n=296) of the women reported consuming milk and other protein rich foods like cheese, paneer, egg etc. during lactation. Among these, significantly higher ($p<0.001$) number of women belonged to OW (46%) and Ob (24.3%) as compared to N and PO.

Table 4.3.2.1 - Special foods consumed during lactation by the women in the four BMI categories; n=387; % (n)

Food		N (n=90)	PO (n=61)	OW (n=156)	Ob (n=80)	% Total (n=387)	P – value
No Special Food	% in sample	11.7 (9)	20.8 (16)	44.2 (34)	23.4 (18)	20.0 (77)	<0.001 (S)
	% within group	10.0 (9)	26.2 (16)	21.8 (34)	22.5 (18)		
Panjiri	% in sample	25.8 (58)	8.4 (19)	49.8 (112)	16.0 (36)	58.2 (225)	<0.001 (S)
	% within group	64.4 (58)	31.1 (19)	71.8 (112)	45.0 (36)		
Milk & other protein rich foods	% in sample	16.9 (50)	12.8 (38)	46.0 (136)	24.3 (72)	76.5 (296)	<0.001 (S)
	% within group	55.6 (50)	62.3 (38)	87.2 (136)	90.0 (72)		
Ghee	% in sample	9.8 (16)	3.1 (5)	47.2 (77)	39.9 (65)	42.2 (163)	<0.001 (S)
	% within group	17.8 (16)	8.2 (5)	49.4 (77)	81.3 (65)		
Fresh fruits/Dry Fruits/ Dalia	% in sample	86.0 (49)	14.0 (8)	0	0	14.7 (57)	<0.001 (S)
	% within group	54.4 (49)	13.1 (8)	0	0		

Parentheses indicate number of subjects; (S) indicates significant.
The level of significance for Chi-square test was taken as $p<0.05$.

Panjeeri was consumed by significantly higher ($p<0.001$) number of women belonging to OW. *Panjeeri* is an energy dense food popularly given to women after childbirth for strength and good lactation.

Consumption of *ghee* after delivery in *dal*, on *chapatti* or in rice was significantly higher ($p<0.001$) for OW (47.2%) and Ob (40.0%) as compared to N (9.8%) and PO (3.1%). The within group data analysis revealed that significantly higher ($p<0.001$) percent women in PO, OW and Ob did not especially include any food in the meals as compared to N. Also, intake of protein rich foods was highest for Ob followed by OW and PO. Also, the consumption of ghee during lactation was highest was Ob (81.3%) as compared to 17.8% in N.

The special foods consumed during lactation was significantly different ($p<0.001$) among the weight categories.

4.3.2.2 Reasons for consuming special foods during lactation

Table 4.3.2.2 gives the data on reasons for consuming special foods during lactation. Significantly higher ($p<0.001$) number of women belonging to OW and N reported consuming special foods, which are galactogogues as compared to women in Ob and PO. On the other hand significantly higher ($p<0.001$) number of women belonging to OW (48.0%) consumed these special foods on advice of elders as compared to women in N, PO and Ob category.

Table 4.3.2.2 - Reasons for consuming special foods during lactation by the women in the four BMI categories; n=310; % (n)

Reasons	N (n=81)	PO (n=45)	OW (n=122)	Ob (n=62)	% Total (n=310)	P – value
Healthy and Galactogogue	28.3 (60)	14.2 (30)	35.4 (75)	22.2 (47)	68.4 (212)	<0.001 (S)
On elder's advice	21.4 (21)	15.3 (15)	48.0 (47)	15.3 (15)	31.6 (98)	<0.001 (S)

Parentheses indicate number of subjects; (S) indicates significant.
The level of significance for Chi-square test was taken as $p<0.05$.

4.3.2.3 Foods avoided during lactation

Percentage of women avoiding certain foods during lactation is given in table 4.3.2.3. The data revealed that 65.4% (n=253) did not avoid any kind of food during lactation. Among these, significantly higher ($p<0.001$) number of women belonged to OW (80.4%). Also, significantly higher ($p<0.001$) percentage of women belonging to N (48.7%) avoided consumption of fried food as compared to women in PO, OW and Ob.

Thus, the kind of foods avoided during lactation was significantly different among weight categories.

Table 4.3.2.3 - Foods avoided during lactation by the women in the four BMI categories; n=387; % (n)

Food	N (n=90)	PO (n=61)	OW (n=156)	Ob (n=80)	% Total (n=387)	P – value
None	16.2 (41)	14.6 (37)	80.4 (123)	20.6 (52)	65.4 (253)	<0.001 (S)
Whole Pulses	24.5 (23)	12.8 (12)	35.1 (33)	27.7 (26)	24.3 (94)	<0.001 (S)
Fried/Heavy Foods	48.7 (36)	16.2 (12)	10.8 (8)	24.3 (18)	19.1 (74)	<0.001 (S)

Parentheses indicate number of subjects; (S) indicates significant.
The level of significance for Chi-square test was taken as $p<0.05$.

4.4 DIETARY PATTERN

People of affluent society are exposed to a great variety of food which often leads to an abundance of intake of energy. At the same time adulthood is the ideal phase of the life cycle for sensitivity to health promotion and disease prevention and women have the potential to shape personal dietary and lifestyle choices and influence those of others. Therefore, food related behaviour and practices were studied in the entire sample (n=387) with respect to type of diet, meal pattern, food preferences, fasting etc. The results have been discussed in the following sections.

4.4.1 Type of diet

The data on type of diet is given in table 4.4.1. It revealed that almost equal number of subjects were distributed in the three types of diet i.e i.e 35% (n=135) of the women were non-vegetarians, 33% (n=127) were vegetarians and 32% were ovo-vegetarians.

Table 4.4.1 - Type of diet of women in the four BMI categories; n=387; % (n)						
Diet	N (n=90)	PO (n=61)	OW (n=156)	Ob (n=80)	% Total (n=387)	P – value
Vegetarian	17.3 (22)	16.5 (21)	40.9 (52)	25.2 (32)	32.8 (127)	0.001 (S)
Ovo-Vegetarian	45.6 (57)	18.4 (23)	36.0 (45)	0	32.3 (125)	
Non vegetarian	8.1 (11)	12.6 (17)	43.7 (59)	35.6 (48)	34.9 (135)	

Parentheses indicate number of subjects; (S) indicates significant.
The level of significance for Chi-square test was taken as $p<0.05$.

Among the non-vegetarians 43.7% were overweight and 35.6% were obese, but only 12.6% were pre-overweight and 8.1% were normal. Thus indicating that majority of the non-vegetarian women were either overweight or obese. Among vegetarian women, 40.9% were overweight and 25.2% were obese. Only 17.3% were normal and 16% were pre-overweight. Whereas, amongst the ovo-vegetarian 45.6% were normal, 36.0% were overweight, 18.4% were pre-overweight and none were obese. Higher percent normal were seen in this group. Type of diet was a significant factor (p=0.001) affecting the weight status of the subjects in the present study.

4.4.2 Frequency of consumption of egg and flesh food

Frequency of consumption of flesh food and eggs is given in table 4.4.2. It revealed that 41.5% of the total non-vegetarian subjects consumed Egg/Flesh foods weekly. Among this group highest consumption was for OW whereas, higher percentage of N subjects reported consuming egg daily or every alternate day.

Table 4.4.2 Frequency of taking flesh/egg products by the women in the four BMI categories; n=260; % (n)						
Frequency	N (n=68)	PO (n=40)	OW (n=104)	Ob (n=48)	% Total (n=260)	p – value
Everyday	32.7 (16)	34.7 (17)	16.3 (8)	16.3 (8)	18.8 (49)	0.001(S)
Every alternate day	43.8 (28)	0	35.9 (23)	20.3 (13)	24.6 (64)	
Once a week	20.4 (22)	21.3 (23)	45.4 (49)	13.0 (14)	41.5 (108)	
Twice a month	0	0	81.2 (13)	18.8 (3)	6.2 (16)	
Once a month	8.7 (2)	0	47.8 (11)	43.5 (10)	8.9 (23)	

Parentheses indicate number of subjects; (S) indicates significant.
The level of significance for Chi-square test was taken as $p<0.05$.

The Chi-square test showed significant difference (p=0.001) among the four BMI categories with respect to the frequency of consumption of egg and flesh foods. Thus, frequency of consumption of flesh/egg was a significant factor affecting the weight status of the subjects in the present study.

4.4.3 Change in type of diet

Table 4.4.3 depicts the type of diet consumed by the subjects previously. A shift from vegetarianism and non-vegetarianism to ovo-vegetarianism was observed.

Table 4.4.3 - Change in type of diet of women in the four BMI categories; n=387; % (n)

Diet		N (n=90)	PO (n=61)	OW (n=156)	Ob (n=80)	% Total (n=387)	P – value
Vegetarian	Earlier	24.3 (33)	15.4 (21)	36.8 (50)	23.5 (32)	35.1 (136)	
	Now	17.3 (22)	16.5 (21)	40.9 (52)	25.2 (32)	32.8 (127)	0.012 (S) (earlier)
Ovo-Vegetarian	Earlier	24.7 (21)	16.5 (14)	52.9 (45)	5.9 (5)	22.0 (85)	
	Now	45.6 (57)	18.4 (23)	36.0 (45)	0	32.3 (125)	
Non vegetarian	Earlier	21.7 (36)	15.7 (26)	36.7 (61)	25.9 (43)	42.9 (166)	0.001 (S) (now)
	Now	8.1 (11)	12.6 (17)	43.7 (59)	35.6 (48)	34.9 (135)	

Parentheses indicate number of subjects; (S) indicates significant.
The level of significance for Chi-square test was taken as $p<0.05$.

There was a significant difference (p=0.012) among the four BMI categories with respect to the previous diet status. Significantly higher (p=0.012) number of women in N category had converted from vegetarianism and non-vegetarianism to ovo-vegetarianism as compared to women in PO, OW and Ob.

4.4.4 Regularity of taking various meals

The meal frequency data of the subjects is given in table 4.4.4. The data revealed that the subjects in all the four BMI categories were consuming eight (8) meals in a day in varying proportions but lunch (90.2%; n=349) and dinner (84.5%; n=327) were consumed by most subjects.

Table 4.4.4 - Percentage women in the four BMI categories taking various meals in a day; n=387; % (n)

Meal		N (n=90)	PO (n=61)	OW (n=156)	Ob (n=80)	% Total (n=387)	P – value
Early Morning	% in sample	20.3 (13)	6.2 (4)	68.8 (44)	4.7 (3)	16.5 (64)	0.001 (S)
	% within group	14.4 (13)	6.6 (4)	28.2 (44)	3.8 (3)		
Breakfast	% in sample	32.1 (90)	21.8 (61)	23.6 (66)	22.5 (63)	72.3 (280)	0.001 (S)
	% within group	100 (90)	100.0 (61)	42.3 (66)	78.8 (63)		
Mid Morning	% in sample	21.6 (36)	18.6 (31)	50.3 (84)	9.6 (18)	43.2 (167)	0.001 (S)
	% within group	40.0 (36)	50.8 (31)	53.9 (84)	22.5 (18)		
Lunch	% in sample	24.6 (86)	13.5 (47)	41.0 (143)	20.9 (73)	90.2 (349)	0.002 (S)
	% within group	95.6 (86)	77.1 (47)	91.7 (143)	91.3 (73)		
After Lunch	% in sample	15.4 (2)	38.5 (5)	23.1 (3)	23.1 (3)	3.4 (13)	0.123 (NS)
	% within group	2.2 (2)	8.2 (5)	1.9 (3)	3.8 (3)		
Evening Tea	% in sample	25.0 (71)	13.0 (37)	44.0 (125)	18.0 (51)	73.4 (284)	0.003 (S)
	% within group	78.9 (71)	60.7 (37)	80.1 (125)	63.8 (51)		
Dinner	% in sample	27.2 (89)	16.5 (54)	39.1 (128)	17.1 (56)	84.5 (327)	0.001 (S)
	% within group	98.9 (89)	88.5 (54)	82.1 (128)	70.0 (56)		
After Dinner	% in sample	10.9 (6)	29.1 (16)	41.8 (23)	18.2 (10)	14.2 (55)	0.009 (S)
	% within group	6.6 (6)	26.2 (16)	14.7 (23)	12.5 (10)		

Parentheses indicate number of subjects; (S) indicates significant; (NS) indicates not significant. The level of significance for Chi-square test was taken as $p<0.05$.

The Chi-square test showed significant difference between the four BMI categories with respect to the consumption of various meals in a day except eating after lunch. Significantly higher (p=0.001) number of women belonging to OW (68.8%; n=44) were eating early morning as compared to just 20.3% in N, 6.2% in PO and 4.7% in Ob.

Breakfast consumption was significantly different (p=0.001) among the women in four BMI categories. The within group analysis revealed that all the N and PO women were taking breakfast as compared to 42.3% of OW and 78.8% of Ob. Also, mid-morning meal consumption was highest for women belonging to OW (50.3%) as compared to women belonging to N (21.6%), PO (18.6%) and Ob (9.6%). The within group analysis also gave similar results.

The percentage women taking lunch was significantly higher for OW (41.0%) as compared to the other three categories. However, within group analysis revealed that significantly higher women of N (95.6%) were taking lunch as compared to women in other three categories. The reason for this difference is that, in the sample OW constitute 40.0% of the total study population, therefore the result of the study population is drifted towards them, but within group data gives a better insight into the habits and behavior of the women in the four categories. There was no significant difference (p=0.123) among the four BMI categories with respect to the post lunch food consumption.

Evening tea was reportedly consumed by 73.4% (n=284) women in the study, of which significantly higher (p=0.003) percentage of women belonged to OW (44.0%; n=125) as compared to just 25% in N, 18% in Ob and 13% in PO.

Consumption of dinner was reported by 84.5% of the study subjects of which significantly higher (p=0.001) percentage belonged to OW. However, within group data revealed that the consumption of dinner was highest by women in N (98.9%) and lowest by women in Ob (70.0%).

After dinner food consumption was significantly higher (p=0.009) for women in OW (41.8%; n=23) as compared to the other three categories. However, the within group analysis revealed that the women in PO (26.2%) were significantly higher (p=0.009) with respect to after dinner meal consumption. Thus regularity of taking meals was a significant factor affecting the weight status of women in the four BMI categories. Significantly higher percentage of N were regularly taking the three main meals as compared to the other three categories.

4.4.5 Eating speed in comparison to others

The data on eating speed in comparison to others has been given in table 4.4.5. It was observed that significantly higher ($p<0.001$) number of women were in OW 48.8% and Ob 26.4% who reported finishing their meals faster in the study sample as compared to just 11.6% in N. The within group analysis revealed that 42.5% of Ob and 40.4% of OW were fast eaters, while 42.6% of PO were slower than others. Thus faster speed of eating in comparison to others had a significant influence on the weight status of the subjects in OW and Ob category in the present study.

Table 4.4.5 - Eating speed of the women in four BMI categories in comparison to others; n=387; % (n)

Eating speed		N (n=90)	PO (n=61)	OW (n=156)	Ob (n=80)	% Total (n=387)	P – value
Faster than others	% in sample	11.6 (15)	13.2 (17)	48.8 (63)	26.4 (34)	33.3 (129)	<0.001 (S)
	% within group	16.7 (15)	27.9 (17)	40.4 (63)	42.5 (34)		
Slower than others	% in sample	34.0 (16)	55.3 (26)	0	10.6 (5)	12.2 (47)	
	% within group	17.8 (16)	42.6(26)	0	6.3 (5)		
Normal with others	% in sample	28.0 (59)	8.5 (18)	44.1 (93)	19.4 (41)	54.5 (211)	
	% within group	65.6 (59)	29.5 (18)	59.6 (93)	51.3 (41)		

Parentheses indicate number of subjects; (S) indicates significant.
The level of significance for Chi-square test was taken as $p<0.05$.

4.4.6 Overeating at meal times

The data on overeating at meal times has been given in table 4.4.6. It was observed that 79.3% women were overeating. Significantly, higher ($p=0.001$) number of women in OW (47.6%), Ob (25.1%) and PO (17.3%) were overeating as compared to just 10% women in N. Within group analysis of data revealed that highest overeating was among Ob women followed by OW and PO. Overeating was a significant factor ($p=0.001$) affecting the weight status of women in the present study.

Table 4.4.6 - Percentage women overeating at meal times in the four BMI categories; n=387; % (n)							
Meal Size		N (n=90)	PO (n=61)	OW (n=156)	Ob (n=80)	% Total (n=387)	P – value
Overeating	% in sample	10.0 (31)	17.3 (53)	47.6 (146)	25.1 (77)	79.3 (307)	0.001 (S)
	% within group	34.4 (31)	86.9 (53)	93.6 (146)	96.3 (77)		
Fixed Meal Size	% in sample	73.8 (59)	10.0 (8)	12.5 (10)	3.8 (3)	20.7 (80)	
	% within group	65.6 (59)	13.1 (8)	6.4 (10)	3.7 (3)		

Parentheses indicate number of subjects; (S) indicates significant;
The level of significance for Chi-square test was taken as $p<0.05$.

4.4.7 Reasons attributed for overeating

The reasons for overeating by the 387 women in the four BMI categories have been given in table 4.4.7.

Table 4.4.7 - Reasons for overeating by the women in the four BMI categories; n=387; % (n)							
Reasons		N (n=90)	PO (n=61)	OW (n=156)	Ob (n=80)	% Total (n=387)	P – value
Hungry	% in sample	22.5 (32)	0	49.3 (70)	28.2 (40)	36.7 (142)	<0.001 (S)
	% within group	35.6 (32)	0	44.9 (70)	50.0 (40)		
Food is appetizing	% in sample	23.6 (37)	12.7 (20)	46.5 (73)	17.2 (27)	40.7 (157)	0.133 (NS)
	% within group	41.1 (37)	32.8 (20)	46.8 (73)	33.8 (27)		
Stress	% in sample	8.8 (6)	13.2 (9)	27.9 (19)	50.0 (34)	17.6 (68)	<0.001 (S)
	% within group	6.6 (6)	14.8 (9)	12.2 (19)	42.5 (34)		
Happy	% in sample	26.7 (8)	20.0 (6)	43.3 (13)	10.0 (3)	7.6 (30)	0.494 (NS)
	% within group	8.9 (8)	9.8 (6)	8.3 (13)	3.4 (3)		
Always overeat	% in sample	20.0 (2)	0	80.0 (8)	0	2.6 (10)	0.05 (NS)
	% within group	2.2 (2)	0	5.1 (8)	0		
Favourite food	% in sample	14.5 (22)	22.4 (34)	42.8 (65)	20.4 (31)	39.3 (152)	0.001 (S)
	% within group	24.4 (22)	55.7 (34)	41.7 (65)	38.8 (31)		

Parentheses indicate number of subjects; (S) indicates significant; (NS) indicates not significant
The level of significance for Chi-square test was taken as $p<0.05$.

It was observed that reasons like hunger, stress and availability of favourite food were significant determinants of overeating.

The data revealed that 36.7% women overate when hungry. Among these significantly higher ($p<0.001$) women were in OW and Ob as compared to N. Also, significantly higher ($p<0.001$) women in Ob were overeating when in stress. Overeating on availability of favourite food was also significantly higher ($p=0.001$) for women in OW as compared to N. Stress was the major contributing factor for overeating among Ob.

4.4.8 Eating in between meals

Eating in between meals was a habit for 46.0% of women in the study sample as shown in table 4.4.8. Among these, significantly higher ($p<0.001$) number of women were in OW (47.2%) and Ob (24.2%) as compared to just 11.8% in N. The within group data revealed that 76.7% of N were eating at fixed time as compared to just 46.0% of OW and Ob. Thus eating in between meals was a significant factor affecting the weight status of women in OW and Ob.

Table 4.4.8 - Percentage women eating in between meals in the four BMI categories; n=387; % (n)

Eating pattern		N (n=90)	PO (n=61)	OW (n=156)	Ob (n=80)	% Total (n=387)	P – value
Eat at fixed meal time only	% in sample	33.0 (69)	14.8 (31)	34.4 (72)	17.7 (37)	54.0 (209)	<0.001 (S)
	% within group	76.7 (69)	50.8 (31)	46.2 (72)	46.3 (37)		
Eat in between meals	% in sample	11.8 (21)	16.9 (30)	47.2 (84)	24.2 (43)	46.0 (178)	
	% within group	23.3 (21)	49.2 (30)	53.8 (84)	53.7 (43)		

Parentheses indicate number of subjects; (S) indicates significant;
The level of significance for Chi-square test was taken as $p<0.05$.

4.4.9 Fasting behaviour

Fasting behaviour of the 387 women was analyzed for frequency, reason and diet consumed while on fast. The results have been tabulated in table 4.4.9.1 to 4.4.9.3.

4.4.9.1 Fasting

Table 4.4.9.1 shows that more than half (56.3%) of study sample reported observing fast. Among these, significantly higher (p<0.001) women were in OW (42.2%) as compared to other three categories. However, within group analysis revealed that significantly higher women of Ob (81.3%) as compared to just 54.4% of N and 59.0% of OW were fasting. Fasting was a significant factor affecting the weight status of women in the study.

Table 4.4.9.1 - Percentage of women observing fasts in the four BMI categories; n=387; % (n)

Fasting		N (n=90)	PO (n=61)	OW (n=156)	Ob (n=80)	% Total (n=387)	P – value
Observe fast	% in sample	22.5 (49)	5.5 (12)	42.2 (92)	29.8 (65)	56.3 (218)	<0.001 (S)
	% within group	54.4 (49)	19.7 (12)	59.0 (92)	81.3 (65)		
Don't fast	% in sample	24.3 (41)	29.0 (49)	37.9 (64)	8.9 (15)	43.7(169)	
	% within group	45.6 (41)	80.3 (49)	41.0 (64)	18.7 (15)		

Parentheses indicate number of subjects; (S) indicates significant;
The level of significance for Chi-square test was taken as p<0.05.

4.4.9.2 Frequency of fasting

Table 4.4.9.2 depicts the frequency of fasting. The data revealed that out of 218 women who reported fasting, 62.4% fasted once a week. Among these, those belonging to OW and Ob were significantly higher (p=0.009) than N. Also, 6.0% women in the sample were fasting twice a week, amongst which, significantly higher (p=0.009) were in Ob. Thus frequency of fasting was significantly different among weight categories.

Table 4.4.9.2 - Frequency of fasting by the women in the four BMI categories; n=218; % (n)						
Frequency	N (n=49)	PO (n=12)	OW (n=92)	Ob (n=65)	% Total (n=218)	P – value
Once a Month	16.3 (8)	10.2 (5)	40.8 (20)	32.7 (16)	22.5 (49)	0.009 (S)
Once a Week	19.9 (27)	5.2 (7)	44.1 (60)	30.9 (42)	62.4 (136)	
Twice a Week	15.4 (2)	0	30.8 (4)	53.8 (7)	6.0 (13)	
Once a Year	60.0 (12)	0	40.0 (8)	0	9.1 (200	

Parentheses indicate number of subjects; (S) indicates significant;
The level of significance for Chi-square test was taken as $p<0.05$.

4.4.9.3 Diet consumed while fasting

The data on pattern of eating on fasting day has been given in table 4.4.9.3. It was observed that significantly higher ($p=0.001$) number of women belonging to Ob (36%) and OW (34.9%) consumed special meal once a day as compared to just 20.9% in N. Special meals included products like *poori, aloo, sabutdana kheer, phirni* and *halwa.* Majority of the women in the study reported abstaining onion, garlic and non-vegetarian food while fasting. Diet consumed while fasting was significantly different among weight categories.

Table 4.4.9.3 Diet consumed while on fast by women in four BMI categories; n=218; % (n)						
Diet	N (n=49)	PO (n=12)	OW (n=92)	Ob (n=65)	% Total (n=218)	P – value
Normal Meal once a day	31.3 (31)	5.1 (5)	44.4 (44)	19.2 (19)	45.4 (99)	0.001 (S)
Special Meal once a day	20.9 (18)	8.1 (7)	34.9 (30)	36.0 (31)	39.5 (86)	
Only Fruit/Water	0	0	54.5 (18)	45.5 (15)	15.1 (33)	

Parentheses indicate number of subjects; (S) indicates significant;
The level of significance for Chi-square test was taken as $p<0.05$.

4.4.10 Changes made in past dietary behaviour

Data in table 4.4.10 revealed that 37.5% women changed their dietary behaviour in last one year. Among these, significantly higher ($p<0.001$) number of women were in Ob (55.2%) as compared just 8.3% in N and 12.4% in PO and 24.1% in OW.

However, within group analysis revealed that all the Ob women had made changes in their dietary behaviour.

Table 4.4.10 - Percentage women who changed their dietary behaviour in the four BMI categories; n=387; % (n)

Dietary Behaviour		N (n=90)	PO (n=61)	OW (n=156)	Ob (n=80)	% Total (n=387)	P – value
Changed	% in sample	8.3 (12)	12.4 (18)	24.1 (35)	55.21 (80)	37.7 (145)	<0.001 (S)
	% within group	13.3 (12)	29.5 (18)	22.4 (35)	100.0 (80)		

Parentheses indicate number of subjects; (S) indicates significant;
The level of significance for Chi-square test was taken as p<0.05.

4.4.11 Reasons for making changes in the dietary behaviour

Reasons for making changes in dietary behaviour have been given in table 4.4.11. The reasons were broadly classified as on advice of doctor/dietician/health clinic/known person successful in losing weight and self imposed. It was observed that significantly higher (p<0.001) women in Ob (59.8%) reported making self imposed dietary changes in comparison to women in other categories.

Table 4.4.11 - Reasons for changing the dietary behaviour by the women in the four BMI categories; n=145; % (n)

Reasons	N (n=12)	PO (n=18)	OW (n=35)	Ob (n=80)	% Total (n=145)	P – value
On advise	0	0	77.8 (14)	22.2 (4)	12.3 (18)	0.169 (NS)
Self Imposed	9.5 (12)	14.2 (18)	16.5 (21)	59.8 (76)	87.7 (127)	<0.001 (S)

Parentheses indicate number of subjects; (S) indicates significant; (NS) indicates not significant
The level of significance for Chi-square test was taken as p<0.05.

4.4.12 Kind of dietary restrictions

The data in table 4.4.12 revealed that the women were either restricting fat or sugar or both. It was observed that significantly higher (p=0.001) percentage of women in Ob were restricting the intake of sugar. Also, significantly higher (p=0.001) percentage of women in OW were restricting intake of fried foods. However, significantly higher (p=0.001) percentage of N were restricting intake of both fat and sugar. Thus the kind dietary restrictions made in the diet by the women in the four categories was significantly different.

Table 4.4.12 - Kind of dietary restrictions by the women in the four BMI categories; n=146; % (n)						
Dietary restrictions	N (n=12)	PO (n=18)	OW (n=35)	Ob (n=80)	% Total (n=145)	P – value
Restricted intake of Fried Foods	0	12.8 (5)	48.78 (19)	38.5 (15	26.9 (39)	0.001 (S)
Restricted intake of Sugar & Sugar Products	0	4.2 (3)	15.3 (11)	80.6 (58)	49.7 (72)	
Restricted intake of both fat and sugar	35.3 (12)	29.4 (10)	14.7 (5)	20.6 (7)	23.4 (34)	
Parentheses indicate number of subjects; (S) indicates significant. The level of significance for Chi-square test was taken as p<0.05.						

4.4.13 Foods especially included in the diet

The data on the variety of foods specially included in the diet has been given in table 4.4.13. The data revealed that significantly higher (p<0.001) number of women in N (33.9%) were especially including food items like sprouts, multigrain atta/breads, fruits and vegetables as compared to just 17.8% in Ob and 16.1% in PO. The intake of these items were comparable for OW but within group analysis revealed that it was lowest amongst all weight categories.

Significantly higher (p<0.001) number of women belonging to OW (39.3%) and N (33.3%) reported including milk and milk products in their diet as compared to just 17.8% and 10.7% in Ob and PO respectively.

Nuts and raisins were included by 18.4% of the women in the study. Among these, significantly higher (p<0.001) number of women belonged to N as compared to other three categories.

Also, 14.7% women in the study reported that they did not especially include anything in their diet. Among these significantly higher (p<0.001) number of women were from OW. Thus foods especially included in the diet were significantly different among weight categories.

Table 4.4.13 - Foods especially included in the diet by the women in four BMI categories; n=387; % (n)

Type of food		N (n=90)	PO (n=61)	OW (n=156)	Ob (n=80)	% Total (n=387)	P – value
Fruits /Salads / Sprouts/ Multi-grain	% in sample	33.9 (61)	16.1 (29)	32.2 (58)	17.8 (32)	46.5 (180)	<0.001 (S)
	% within group	67.8 (61)	47.5 (29)	37.2 (58)	40.0 (32)		
Milk / Curd / Cheese	% in sample	33.3 (84)	10.7 (27)	39.3 (99)	17.8 (45)	65.1 (252)	<0.001 (S)
	% within group	93.3 (84)	44.3 (27)	63.5 (99)	56.3 (45)		
Almonds / Walnut	% in sample	53.5 (38)	14.1 (10)	7.0 (5)	25.4 (18)	18.4 (71)	<0.001 (S)
	% within group	42.2 (38)	16.4 (10)	3.2 (5)	22.5 (18)		
Do not include anything especially	% in sample	0	12.3 (7)	61.4 (35)	26.3 (15)	14.5 (57)	<0.001 (S)
	% within group	0	11.5 (7)	22.4 (35)	18.8 (15)		

Parentheses indicate number of subjects; (S) indicates significant;
The level of significance for Chi-square test was taken as $p<0.05$.

4.4.14 Snacking Behaviour

In the present study the snacking behaviour of the 387 women was analysed with respect to the frequency of consumption of snacks and preference for variety of snacks.

4.4.14.1 Frequency of eating snacks

The data on frequency of snack consumption has been given in table 4.4.14.1. It was observed that almost 73% women were consuming some kind of snack daily. In this group significantly higher ($p<0.001$) number of women were in OW (47.9%) as compared to just 22.3% in Ob, 16.0% in N and 13.8% in PO. However, the within group data revealed that as compared to 50.0% in N, significantly higher ($p<0.001$) women in PO (63.9%), OW (86.5%) and Ob (78.6%) were eating snack daily. Thus higher frequency of consuming snacks was a significant factor affecting the weight status of women.

Table 4.4.14.1 - Frequency of snack consumption among women in the four BMI categories; n=387; % (n)

Frequency		N (n=90)	PO (n=61)	OW (n=156)	Ob (n=80)	% Total (n=387)	P – value
Eat Daily	% in sample	16.0 (45)	13.8 (39)	47.9 (135)	22.3 (63)	72.9 (282)	<0.001 (S)
	% within group	50.0 (45)	63.9 (39)	86.5 (135)	78.6 (63)		
Eat Occasionally	% in sample	42.9 (45)	21.0 (22)	20.0 (21)	16.2 (17)	27.1 (105)	
	% within group	50.0 (45)	36.1 (22)	13.5 (21)	21.3 (17)		

Parentheses indicate number of subjects; (S) indicates significant;
The level of significance for Chi-square test was taken as $p<0.05$.

4.4.14.2 Type of snacks consumed

It is not only the frequency of snacking but also the type of snacks consumed that affects the weight status. The women gave a wide list of snacks being consumed by them, which were broadly divided as *potato wafer, bhujia and namkeen, biscuits, cakes* and *pastries, samaso/pakora* and fruits/salads. The data on snack consumption has been given in table 4.4.14.2. The table reflects that preference for energy dense snacks like *potato wafers, namkeen, biscuits, samosa and pakora* was significantly higher ($p<0.001$) for women in OW and Ob as compared to PO and N. However, the detailed analysis revealed that consumption of potato wafers was highest for OW (50.6%) and least for N (12.0%). Similarly, consumption of *bhujia* and other *namkeens* was highest among OW (44.8%) and again least among N.

Table 4.4.14.2 - Types of snacks consumed by women in the four BMI categories; n=387; % (n)						
Type of snacks	N (n=90)	PO (n=61)	OW (n=156)	Ob (n=80)	% Total (n=387)	P – value
Potato Wafers	12.0 (10)	16.9 (14)	50.6 (42)	20.5 (17)	21.5 (83)	<0.001 (S)
Bhujia & Namkeen	16.1 (23)	18.9 (27)	44.8 (64)	20.2 (29)	37.0(143)	<0.001 (S)
Biscuits	18.2 (23)	24.6 (31)	45.2 (57)	11.9 (15)	32.6 (126)	<0.001 (S)
Cakes & Pastries	39.1 (9)	17.4 (4)	30.5 (7)	13.0 (3)	5.9 (23)	0.07 (NS)
Samosa & Pakora	20.0 (12)	6.7 (4)	35.0 (21)	38.3 (23)	15.5 (60)	<0.001 (S)
Fruits & Salads	19.9 (26)	6.9 (9)	36.6 (48)	36.6 (48)	33.9 (131)	<0.001 (S)

Parentheses indicate number of subjects; (S) indicates significant; (NS) indicates not significant. The level of significance for Chi-square test was taken as $p<0.05$.

Consumption of biscuits was again highest for OW (45.2%) but least among Ob (11.9%). Intake of cakes and pastries was reported by just 5.9% women and there was no significant difference ($p=0.07$) among the four BMI categories. Although 15.5% women reported consuming *samosa* and *pakora*, but it was significantly higher ($p<0.001$) for women belonging to Ob (38.3%) and OW (35.0%) as compared to just 20.0% and 6.7% for N and PO respectively. Consumption of fruits and salads as snacks was also significantly higher ($p<0.001$) for women in OW and Ob as compared to N and PO. Thus, in the present study, intake of variety of snacks was significantly different among weight categories.

4.4.15 Convenience foods

In today's world not only the availability but also the consumption of convenience foods has increased due to the swiftness associated with it. However, most of these foods contain high percentage of fat and sugar, thus making them calorie dense. Therefore, in the present study the pattern of consumption of convenience foods along with the type popularly consumed were studied amongst the study population. Convenience foods for the women in the study included packet soups, instant noodles and pasta, frozen snacks and ready mixes of South India and North India dishes.

4.4.15.1 Consumption of convenience foods

The data on consumption of convenience foods has been given in table 4.4.15.1. The data revealed that 47.6% women were using/consuming convenience foods. In this group significantly higher ($p<0.001$) number of women were in OW (33.2%) as compared to just 17.9% in N. However, the within group data revealed that the consumption of convenience foods was highest among PO, followed by Ob. Thus, consumption of convenience foods significantly differed among weight categories.

Table 4.4.15.1 - Consumption of convenience foods among women in the four BMI category; n=387; % (n)

Convenience foods	N (n=90)	PO (n=61)	OW (n=156)	Ob (n=80)	% Total (n=387)	P – value
% in sample	17.9 (33)	23.4 (43)	33.2 (61)	25.5 (47)	47.6 (184)	<0.001(S)
% within group	36.7 (33)	70.5 (43)	39.1 (61)	58.8 (47)		

Parentheses indicate number of subjects; (S) indicates significant;
The level of significance for Chi-square test was taken as $p<0.05$.

4.4.15.2 Frequency of consumption of convenience foods

Table 4.4.15.2 depicts the frequency of consumption of convenience foods. The frequency data revealed that out of 184 subjects consuming convenience foods, 50.0% were consuming such foods once a week. In this group significantly higher ($p<0.001$) number of women belonged to OW (35.9%) and Ob (28.3%) as compared to just 15.2% in N. Frequency of consumption of convenience foods was significant different among weight categories.

Table 4.4.15.2 - Frequency of consumption of convenience foods by the women in the four BMI categories; n=184; % (n)

Frequency	N (n=33)	PO (n=43)	OW (n=61)	Ob (n=47)	% Total (n=184)	P – value
Everyday	0	0	85.7 (12)	14.3 (2)	7.6 (14)	<0.001 (S)
Once a Week	15.2 (14)	20.7 (19)	35.9 (33)	28.3 (26)	50.0 (92)	
Once a Month	37.5 (9)	0	37.5 (9)	25.0 (6)	13.0 (24)	
Occasionally	18.5 (10)	44.4 (24)	13.0 (7)	24.1 (13)	29.4 (54)	

Parentheses indicate number of subjects; (S) indicates significant;
The level of significance for Chi-square test was taken as $p<0.05$.

4.4.15.3 Type of convenience foods consumed

The popularly consumed convenience foods were soups and juices, North Indian dishes, noodles and pastas, frozen snacks like cutlets, french-fries, samosa etc., and South Indian mix like idly, dosa, upma etc. The variety of convenience foods used has been tabulated in table 4.4.15.3. Amongst the variety of convenience foods, 56.0% reported preference for instant noodles and pasta. In this group significantly higher ($p<0.001$) number of women belonged to OW (32.1%) and Ob (30.1%) as compared to just 12.6% in N.

Table 4.4.15.3 - Type of convenience foods consumed by women in the four BMI categories; n=184; % (n)

Type	N (n=33)	PO (n=43)	OW (n=61)	Ob (n=47)	% Total (n=184)	P – value
Soups & Juices	22.8 (23)	31.7 (32)	35.6 (36)	9.9 (10)	54.9 (101)	<0.001 (S)
North Indian Dishes	18.2 (6)	0	33.3 (11)	48.5 (16)	17.9 (33)	<0.001 (S)
Noodles & Pasta	12.6 (13)	25.2 (26)	32.1 (33)	30.1 (31)	56.0 (103)	<0.001 (S)
Frozen Foods	13.6 (4)	0	26.7 (8)	60.0 (18)	16.3 (30)	<0.001 (S)
South Indian Mix	1.5 (1)	12.3 (8)	44.6 (29)	41.5 (27)	35.3 (65)	<0.001 (S)

Parentheses indicate number of subjects; (S) indicates significant;
The level of significance for Chi-square test was taken as $p<0.05$

Soups and juices were reportedly consumed by 54.9% women. Among these significantly higher ($p<0.001$) number of women belong to OW (35.6%) and PO (35.7%) as compared to 22.8% in N and 9.9% in Ob.

Also South Indian mixes were consumed by significantly higher ($p<0.001$) number of women belonging to OW (44.6%) and Ob (41.5%) as compared to just 1.5% in N.

Similarly consumption of North Indian dishes and frozen snacks was significantly higher ($p<0.001$) for women belonging to Ob as compared to other three categories.

Thus the type of convenience foods consumed had a significant effect on the weight status of women in OW and Ob categories.

4.4.16 Consumption of sugar in a cup of tea/coffee

Table 4.4.16 depicts the data on consumption of sugar in a day by the women in the four BMI categories. It was observed that significantly higher ($p<0.001$) number of women in OW were consuming sugar in greater proportion than women in N, PO and Ob. The consumption of sugar by the women in N was comparable to that of Ob. Consumption of sugar was significantly different among weight categories.

Table 4.4.16 - Consumption of sugar in a cup of tea/coffee by the women in the four BMI categories; n=387; % (n)

Sugar Consumption	N (n=90)	PO (n=61)	OW (n=156)	Ob (n=80)	% Total (n=387)	P – value
No sugar	37.1 (13)	25.7(9)	37.1 (13)	0	9.0 (35)	<0.001 (S)
One tea spoon	24.1 (65)	17.8 (48)	34.1 (92)	24.1 (65)	69.8 (270)	
Two tea spoons	14.6 (12)	4.9 (4)	62.2 (51)	18.3 (15)	21.2 (82)	

Parentheses indicate number of subjects; (S) indicates significant.
The level of significance for Chi-square test was taken as $p<0.05$.

4.4.17 Consumption of soft drinks

The term 'Soft drink' in the study includes sweetened carbonated drinks, fruit juices, lemonade, Ice tea, squash, sherbet and lassi. Table 4.4.17 (a) depicts the preference of the women in the study sample for various types of soft drinks.

It was observed that consumption of carbonated soft drinks was highest for OW (47.5%) and least for N (5.8%). But within group data highlighted that all the eighty women in Ob (100%) preferred consuming carbonated beverages. Fruit juice was a popular drink among all women, but its consumption was significantly higher ($p<0.001$) for OW (40.4%) as compared to other three categories. However, within group preference data revealed that significantly higher ($p<0.001$) women Ob (97.5%) and PO (96.7%) preferred consuming fruit juice as compared to OW (87.2%) and N (71.1%). Consumption of lemonade was again significantly higher ($p<0.001$) for OW and Ob as compared to N, but within group analysis showed that all women in PO and Ob were taking lemonade. Consumption of squashes and sherbets was significantly higher ($p<0.001$) for OW (40.2%) and PO (22.6%) as compared to N (16.7%) and Ob

(20.5%). Significantly higher (p<0.001) number of women in OW (47.0%) reported taking sweetened lassi.

Table 4.4.17 (a) - Preference for various soft drinks by the women in the four BMI categories; n=387; % (n)

Soft drinks		N (n=90)	PO (n=61)	OW (n=156)	Ob (n=80)	% Total (n=387)	P – value
Carbonated	% in sample	5.8(15)	15.8(41)	47.5(123)	30.9(80)	66.9(259)	<0.001 (S)
	% within group	16.7(15)	67.2(41)	78.8(123)	100.0(80)		
Fruit Juice	% in sample	19.0(64)	17.5(59)	40.4(136)	23.1(78)	87.1(337)	<0.001 (S)
	% within group	71.1(64)	96.7(59)	87.2(136)	97.5(78)		
Lemonade / Ice-tea	% in sample	16.6(50)	20.2(61)	36.8(111)	26.5(80)	78.0(302)	<0.001 (S)
	% within group	55.6(50)	100.0(61)	71.2(111)	100.0(80)		
Squashes and sherbet	% in sample	16.7 (39)	22.6 (53)	40.2 (94)	20.5 (48)	60.5(234)	<0.001 (S)
	% within group	43.3 (39)	86.9 (53)	60.3 (94)	60.0 (48)		
Lassi	% in sample	21.3 (68)	9.4 (30)	47.0 (150)	22.3 971)	82.4(319)	<0.001 (S)
	% within group	75.6 (68)	49.2 (30)	96.2 (150)	88.6 (71)		

Parentheses indicate number of subjects; (S) indicates significant.
The level of significance for Chi-square test was taken as p<0.05.

Table 4.4.17(b) reveals the data on frequency of consumption of these soft drinks in a day by the women in the study. It was observed that significantly higher (p<0.001) number of women in OW and Ob category were taking soft drinks at a greater frequency i.e. twice in a day or more than that as compared to women in N and PO.

Thus, not only the consumption of soft drinks, but also its frequency of consumption is a significant factor affecting the weight status of the women in the study.

Table 4.4.17 (b) - Frequency of consumption of soft drinks in a day by the women in the four BMI categories; n=387; % (n)						
Frequency	N (n=90)	PO (n=61)	OW (n=156)	Ob (n=80)	% Total (n=387)	P – value
None	78.6 (22)	0	21.4 (6)	0	7.2 (28)	<0.001 (S)
Once	30.8 (48)	22.4 (35)	34.6 (54)	12.2 (19)	40.3 (156)	
Twice	13.4 (20)	13.4 (20)	42.3 (63)	30.9 (46)	38.5 (149)	
More than two times	0	11.1 (6)	61.1 (33)	27.8 (15)	13.9 (54)	

Parentheses indicate number of subjects; (S) indicates significant.
The level of significance for Chi-square test was taken as $p<0.05$.

Table 4.4.18 - Mean monthly household consumption of various types of fats & oils by the women in the four BMI categories; (n=387) (mean ± SD with range)						
Kinds of Oils	N (n=90)	PO (n=61)	OW (n=156)	Ob (n=80)	Total (n=387)	P – value
Refined Oil (l)	2.8 ± 1.11^{a} (1.0-5.0)	2.4 ± 0.81^{a1} (1.0-5.0)	3.11 ± 1.39 (1.0-5.6)	3.1 ± 1.24 (1.0-5.0)	2.9 ± 1.24 (1.0-5.6)	<0.001 (S)
Vanaspati	0	0	0	0	0	0
Desi Ghee (g)	508.8 ± 280.7^{b} (100-1500)	404.8 ± 152.8^{b1} (250-1000)	766.5 ± 354^{b2} (100-2000)	1154.7 ± 702.6 (500-3000)	703.3 ± 463.8 (100-3000)	<0.001 (S)
Mustard Oil (ml)	1111 ± 1359^{c} (250-5000)	668.2 ± 382.4^{c1} (200-1500)	693 ± 461.9^{c2} (50-2000)	1129 ± 093.7 (500-5000)	864.3 ± 866.5 (50-500)	0.024 (S)
Butter (g)	336.4 ± 176.2^{d} (100-500)	400.0 ± 159.5 (100-500)	443.7 ± 135.6^{d1} (100-500)	404.5 ± 132.2 (100-500)	399.6 ± 156.5 (100-500)	<0.001 (S)

The level of significance for ANOVA was taken as $p<0.05$; (S) indicates significant.

Intake of refined oil; (ANOVA)
[a] - N < OW, Ob; [a1] - PO < OW, Ob

Intake of desi ghee; (ANOVA)
[b] - N < OW, Ob; [b1] - PO < OW, Ob; [b2] - OW < Ob

Intake of mustard oil; (ANOVA)
[c] - N > PO, OW; [c1] - PO < Ob; [c2] - OW < Ob

Intake of butter; (ANOVA)
[d] - N < PO, OW, Ob; [d1] - OW > PO, Ob

4.4.18 Monthly household consumption of fats and oils

Table 4.4.18 depicts the data on mean monthly household consumption of various fats and oils by the women in the four BMI categories. It was observed that mean monthly household consumption of refined oil was signif5icantly higher ($p<0.001$) for women in OW and Ob as compared to N and PO.

The monthly consumption of desi ghee was significantly higher ($p<0.001$) for Ob households as compared to that of the other three categories. The mean monthly household consumption of mustard oil was significantly higher ($P=0.024$) for N and Ob in comparison to PO and OW. The mean monthly consumption of butter was significantly higher ($p<0.001$) for OW as compared to the other three categories.

It was observed that the mean monthly intake of variety of fats and oils was more in Ob households as compared to the other three. Thus, indicating that the amount of fat and oil used per month in a house is a significant factor affecting the weight status of women in the study.

4.4.19 Frequency of consumption of fried food products

The frequency of consumption of fried food products has been depicted in table 4.4.19. It was observed that frequency of consumption was significantly higher ($p<0.001$) for women belonging to OW and Ob as compared to PO and N for once a week. However, 39.0% consumed fired food products and 25.1% completely avoided.

Table 4.4.19 - Frequency of consumption of Fried food products by the women in four BMI categories; n=387; % (n)

Frequency	N (n=90)	PO (n=61)	OW (n=156)	Ob (n=80)	% Total (n=387)	P – value
Twice a Week	26.3 (10)	0	73.7 (28)	0	9.8 (38)	<0.001 (S)
Once a Week	9.9 (10)	18.8 (9)	33.7 (34)	37.6 (38)	26.1 (101)	
Occasionally	27.2 (41)	25.2 (38)	39.7 (60)	7.9 (12)	39.0 (151)	
Avoid Completely	29.9 (29)	4.1 (4)	35.1 (34)	30.9 (30)	25.1 (97)	

Parentheses indicate number of subjects; (S) indicates significant.
The level of significance for Chi-square test was taken as $p<0.05$.

4.4.20 Milk Consumption

Milk consumption of the study subjects was studied with respect to the consumption/day and the type of milk consumed.

4.4.20.1 Milk consumption per day

The data on milk consumption has been given in table 4.4.20.1. The data revealed that 70.8% women in the study sample consumed milk at least once a day. Among these, significantly higher (p=0.013) were in OW (42.3%) as compared to 21.9% in Ob, 19.7% in N and 16.1% in PO. However, the within group analysis revealed that significantly higher (p=0.013) number of women of PO, OW, Ob were consuming milk as compared to that of N.

Also 21.0% women reported consuming milk twice a day. In this group significantly higher women were in N and Ob as compared to PO and Ob. But, within group analysis revealed that more number of N and PO women were taking milk twice daily as compared to OW and Ob.

Table 4.4.20.1 - Frequency of milk consumed per day by the women in the four BMI categories; n=387; % (n)

<table>
<tr><th colspan="2">Frequency of Milk</th><th>N (n=90)</th><th>PO (n=61)</th><th>OW (n=156)</th><th>Ob (n=80)</th><th>% Total (n=387)</th><th>P – value</th></tr>
<tr><td rowspan="2">Once</td><td>% in sample</td><td>19.7 (54)</td><td>16.1 (44)</td><td>42.3 (116)</td><td>21.9 (60)</td><td rowspan="2">70.8 (274)</td><td rowspan="6">0.013 (S)</td></tr>
<tr><td>% within group</td><td>60.0 (54)</td><td>72.1 (44)</td><td>74.4 (116)</td><td>75.0 (60)</td></tr>
<tr><td rowspan="2">Twice</td><td>% in sample</td><td>33.3 (27)</td><td>21.0 (17)</td><td>30.9 (25)</td><td>14.8 (12)</td><td rowspan="2">21.0 (81)</td></tr>
<tr><td>% within group</td><td>30.0 (27)</td><td>27.9 (17)</td><td>16.0 (25)</td><td>15.0 (12)</td></tr>
<tr><td rowspan="2">Not at all</td><td>% in sample</td><td>28.1 (9)</td><td>0</td><td>46.9 (15)</td><td>25.0 (8)</td><td rowspan="2">8.3 (32)</td></tr>
<tr><td>% within group</td><td>10.0 (9)</td><td>0</td><td>9.6 (15)</td><td>10.0 (8)</td></tr>
</table>

Parentheses indicate number of subjects; (S) indicates significant.
The level of significance for Chi-square test was taken as p<0.05.

4.4.20.2 Type of milk consumed

There was a wide variety in the type of milk consumed as observed from table 4.4.20.2. The various milks consumed were toned, double toned, full cream, homogenized, *gawala* cow milk and *gawala* buffalo milk.

The 355 women who reported consuming milk, 63.4% (n=225) reported consuming toned milk. Amongst these, significantly higher (p= 0.001) number of women belonged to OW (41.8%) as compared to 21.8% to N, 19.6% to Ob and just 16.9% to PO.

A small percentage of women (2.5%) were consuming double toned milk, of which 55.6%belonged to PO and remaining 44.4% to Ob and none to N and PO.

Also, 24.0% women reported consuming full cream milk, of which significantly higher (p=0.001) women were in N and Ob as compared to PO and N.

Mother dairy's homogenized milk was consumed by 7.6% women of which significantly higher (p=0.001) number of women belonged to N, PO and OW as compared to Ob.

Thus the type of milk consumed by women in the four BMI categories was a significant factor affecting their weight status.

Table 4.4.20.2 - Types of milk consumed by the women in the four BMI categories; n=355; % (n)

Type of Milk	N (n=81)	PO (n=61)	OW (n=141)	Ob (n=72)	% Total (n=355)	P – value
Toned	21.8 (49)	16.9 (38)	41.8 (94)	19.6 (44)	63.4 (225)	0.001 (S)
Double Toned	0	55.6 (5)	0	44.4 (4)	2.5 (9)	
Full Cream	32.9 (28)	12.9 (11)	24.7 (21)	29.4 (25)	24.0 (85)	
Homogenised Milk	33.3 (9)	25.9 (7)	33.3 (9)	7.4 (2)	7.6 (27)	
Gawala Cow Milk	100.0 (6)	0	0	0	1.7 (6)	
Gawala Buffalo Milk	0	0	0	100.0 (3)	0.9 (3)	

Parentheses indicate number of subjects; (S) indicates significant.
The level of significance for Chi-square test was taken as p<0.05.

4.4.20.3 Consumption of Milk Fat

The data on consumption of milk fat, i.e. malai in common parlance has been given in table 4.4.20.3. It was observed that 71.0% women were consuming malai along with milk. Amongst these significantly higher (p=0.003) women were in OW (35.7%) as compared to the other three categories.

Table 4.4.20.3 - Consumption of milk fat by the women in the four BMI categories; n=355; % (n)

Consumption	N (n=81)	PO (n=61)	OW (n=141)	Ob (n=72)	% Total (n=355)	P – value
Fat Consumed	22.2 (56)	22.2 (56)	35.7 (90)	19.8 (50)	71.0 (252)	0.003 (S)
Fat Removed	24.3 (25)	4.9 (5)	49.5 (51)	21.4 (22)	29.0 (103)	

Parentheses indicate number of subjects; (S) indicates significant.
The level of significance for Chi-square test was taken as p<0.05.

4.4.21 Consumption of fruits and vegetables

The consumption of fruits and vegetables by the women in the study sample was studied with respect to the servings of fruits / vegetables consumed in a day. The data has been given in Table 4.4.21. It was observed that the intake of fruits/vegetables per day was not significantly different (p=0.121) for the women in N, PO, OW and Ob.

Table 4.4.21 - Servings of fruits/vegetables consumed per day by the women in the four BMI categories; n=387; % (n)

Servings	N (n=90)	PO (n=61)	OW (n=156)	Ob (n=80)	% Total (n=387)	P – value
At least one	0	0	100.0 (8)	0	2.1 (8)	0.121 (NS)
Two	23.2 (43)	14.1 (26)	42.2 (78)	20.5 (38)	47.8 (185)	
More than two	24.2 (47)	18.0 (35)	36.1 (70)	21.6 (42)	50.1 (194)	

Parentheses indicate number of subjects; (NS) indicates not significant.

The level of significance for Chi-square test was taken as p<0.05.

4.5 EATING OUT PATTERN

Eating out pattern of the study subjects was analysed for frequency of eating out, the food choices made while eating out, typical meal taken when at home, frequency of attending social gatherings and food preference in these gatherings.

4.5.1 Frequency of eating out

The data on frequency of eating out has been given in table 4.5.1. It was observed that outside food was most frequently consumed once a week by 59.4% women. Among these, significantly higher ($p<0.001$) number of women were in OW (53.0%) as compared to just 18.3% in PO, 15.2% in N and 13.5% in Ob. Also, eight women each in OW and Ob category reported eating out twice a week as compared to none in N and PO. However, 12 women in N reported eating out daily as compared to just one in Ob and none in PO and OW. The data also revealed that 33.1% women were eating out fortnightly or once a month. In this group significantly higher ($p<0.001$) number of women belong to N and Ob as compared to OW and PO. Thus the frequency of eating out was significantly different among weight categories.

Table 4.5.1 - Frequency of eating out by the women in four BMI categories; n=387; % (n)

Frequency	N (n=90)	PO (n=61)	OW (n=156)	Ob (n=80)	% Total (n=387)	P – value
Once a Week	15.2 (35)	18.3 (42)	53.0 (122)	13.5 (31)	59.4 (230)	<0.001 (S)
Twice a Week	0	0	50.0 (8)	50.0 (8)	4.1 (16)	
Daily	92.3 (12)	0	0	7.7 (1)	3.4 (13)	
Fortnightly / once a month	33.6 (43)	14.8 (19)	20.3 (26)	31.3 (40)	33.1(128)	

Parentheses indicate number of subjects; (S) indicates significant.
The level of significance for Chi-square test was taken as $p<0.05$.

4.5.2 Food preference on eating out

It is not only the frequency of eating out, which affects the weight status, but also the choice of food preferred for eating. Therefore, in the present study the food preference of the subjects with respect to various foods as well as whether these foods constituted part of the main meals or in between meals was analysed. The results have been tabulated in Table 4.5.2.1 and 4.5.2.2.

4.5.2.1 Food preference while eating out

Food preferences while eating out were broadly classified as fast foods, North Indian/Mughlai, South Indian and snacks and desserts. Fast foods included items like pizza, burger, pasta, noodles, sandwich etc. North Indian/Mughlai category included items like *chole bhature, tandoori roti, parantha* with subzi/vegetarian or non-vegetarian curries. South Indian food included all items of southern and coastal cuisine. Snacks and desserts category included items like *samosa, tikki, dahi bhalla, bhel puri, cutlets, kababs* etc. It also included ice-creams, kulfi and other Indian sweets.

Table 4.5.2.1 gives the data on the preferences of women in the four BMI categories while eating out.

Table 4.5.2.1 - Preference of food by the women in four BMI categories while eating out; n=387; % (n)

Food Preference		N (n=90)	PO (n=61)	OW (n=156)	Ob (n=80)	% Total (n=387)	P – value
Fast Foods	% in sample	16.5 (41)	12.9 (32)	47.0 (117)	23.7 (59)	64.3 (249)	<0.001 (S)
	% within group	45.6 (41)	52.5 (32)	75.0 (117)	73.8 (59)		
North Indian / Mughlai	% in sample	13.7 (29)	17.0 (36)	52.4 (111)	17.0 (36)	54.8 (212)	<0.001 (S)
	% within group	32.2 (29)	59.0 (36)	71.2 (111)	45.0 (36)		
South Indian	% in sample	27.1 (62)	8.7 (20)	44.5 (102)	19.7 (45)	59.2 (229)	<0.001 (S)
	% within group	68.9 (62)	32.8 (20)	65.4 (102)	56.3 (45)		
Snacks and Desserts	% in sample	19.0 (45)	14.8 (35)	41.4 (98)	24.9 (59)	61.2 (237)	0.001 (S)
	% within group	50.0 (45)	57.4 (35)	62.8 (98)	73.8 (59)		

Parentheses indicate number of subjects; (S) indicates significant.
The level of significance for Chi-square test was taken as p<0.05.

It was observed that 64.3% women in the study preferred eating variety of fast foods while eating out. Among these, significantly higher ($p<0.001$) number of women belong to OW (47.0%) as compared to just 23.7% in Ob, 16.5 % in N and 12.9% in PO. However, within group analysis revealed that preference for fast food was highest in OW followed closely by Ob. Also, 59.2% women reported preference for South Indian food. In this group significantly higher ($p<0.001$) number of women belonged to OW as compared to women in other three categories.

The within group data with respect to the preference for South India food revealed that the preference for this food was highest in N when eating out. North Indian and Mughlai food was preferred by 54.8% women. Among these, significantly higher ($p<0.001$) were in OW (52.4%) as compared to just 17.0% each in PO and Ob and 13.7% in N. The within group analysis also supported this result. The preference for snacks and desserts was reported by 61.2% of the study subjects, of which significantly higher ($p<0.001$) belong to OW. However, the within group data revealed that the preference for snacks and desserts was highest in Ob as compared to the other three categories.

4.5.2.2 Eating out for main meals or snacks

The data for eating out for meals or snacks has been given in Table 4.5.2.2. It was observed that there was no significant difference ($p=0.248$) among the women in the four BMI categories with respect to eating out for main meals.

Table 4.5.2.2 - Percentage women eating out for main meals or snacks in four BMI categories; n=387; % (n)

Preference	N (n=90)	PO (n=61)	OW (n=156)	Ob (n=80)	% Total (n=387)	P – value
Main Meals	25.2 (53)	13.8 (29)	35.8 (75)	25.2 (53)	54.3 (210)	0.248 (NS)
Snacks (in between meals)	21.2 (33)	17.9 (28)	45.5 (71)	15.4 (24)	40.3 (156)	<0.001 (S)
Sometimes meals and sometimes snacks	19.0 (4)	19.0 (4)	47.6 (10)	14.3 (3)	5.4 (21)	0.142 (NS)

Parentheses indicate number of subjects; (S) indicates significant; (NS) indicates not significant
The level of significance for Chi-square test was taken as $p<0.05$.

However, there was a significant difference among the women when analysed for eating out for snacks. Significantly higher ($p<0.001$) women in OW (44.9%) were eating out for snacks as compared to just 21.2% in N, 17.9% in PO and 16.0% in Ob. Thus eating out for snacks was significantly different among weight categories.

4.5.3 Food preference when staying at home

Food preference of the subjects when eating at home was analysed with respect to type of food as well as whether the food was homemade or ordered from outside. The data has been given in tables 4.5.3.1 and 4.5.3.2.

4.5.3.1 Type of food eaten at home

Table 4.5.3.1 gives the data on types of food eaten by the 387 women while staying at home. It was observed that 70% of the women in the study were eating chapatti with *subzi* and *dal* or curry. In this group, significantly lesser ($p=0.01$) number of women belong to Ob (20.3%) as compared to 39.9% in OW and 25.5% in N. Also, 16.6% women in four BMI categories reported consuming *parantha* with either curd or *pickle*.

Table 4.5.3.1 - Preference of food when eating at home by the women in four BMI categories; n=387; % (n)

Preference	N (n=90)	PO (n=61)	OW (n=156)	Ob (n=80)	% Total (n=387)	P – value
Chapati and subzi ± dal/curry	25.5 (69)	14.4 (39)	39.9 (108)	20.3 (5)	70.0 (271)	0.01 (S)
Plain Rice and Dal/Curry	33.2 (76)	21..4 (49)	26.6 (61)	18.8 (43)	59.2 (229)	0.016 (S)
Parantha with pickle/curd	17.2 (11)	15.6 (10)	46.9 (30)	20.3 (13)	16.6 (64)	0.01 (S)
Pulao	31.8 (14)	18.2 (8)	11.4 (5)	38.6 (17)	11.4 (44)	0.01 (S)
Salad / Fruit	26.2 (75)	16.4 (47)	37.1 (106)	20.3 (58)	73.9 (286)	0.061 (S)
Any Other	31.0 (90)	14.0 (41)	33.8 (98)	21.0 (61)	74.9 (290)	<0.001 (S)

Parentheses indicate number of subjects; (S) indicates significant.
The level of significance for Chi-square test was taken as $p<0.05$.

Among these significantly higher (p=0.01) number of women belonged to OW as compared to other three categories. Plain rice with *dal* or curry was reportedly consumed by 59.2% women. In this group, significantly higher (p=0.016) number of women were in N (33.2%) as compared to just 26.6% in OW, 21.4% in PO and 18.8% in Ob. *Pulao* as a meal was consumed by 11.4% women, of which significantly higher (p=0.01) number of women were in Ob as compared to other three categories. Almost 74.0% women consumed salad and fruit when at home. Among this group, significantly higher (p=0.061) number of women belonged to OW (37.1%) as compared to 26.6% in N, 20.3% in Ob and just 16.4% in PO. It was observed that 75.0% of women in the study sample reported consuming multigrain flour, boiled/baked vegetarian / non-vegetarian products, boiled *channa*, roasted *papad* with soup etc. In this group, significantly higher (p<0.001) women belonged to OW (33.8%) and N (31.0%) as compared to just 21.0% in Ob and 14.0% in PO.

4.5.3.2 Preference for home cooked food versus ordering from outside while at home

Data in table 4.5.3.2 revealed that 84.0% women preferred eating home cooked meals when eating at home. In this group, significantly lower (p<0.001) women belonged to Ob as compared to other three categories. Although just 5.4% women reported ordering food from outside, but in this group all were in OW (61.9%) and Ob (38.1%). Supplementing home cooked food with outside food was also reported by 10.6% women. Among these women, significantly higher (p<0.001) number of women belonged to Ob as compared to other three categories.

Table 4.5.3.2 - Preference for home cooked food versus ordered food or both by the women in the four BMI categories; n=387; % (n)

Preference	N (n=90)	PO (n=61)	OW (n=156)	Ob (n=80)	% Total (n=387)	P – value
Only home cooked	24.0 (78)	17.5 (57)	40.9 (133)	17.5 (57)	84.0 (325)	<0.001 (S)
Order from Outside	0	0	61.9 (13)	38.1 (8)	5.4 (21)	
Supplement home food with Outside Food	29.3 (12)	9.8 (4)	24.4 (10)	36.6 (15)	10.6 (41)	

Parentheses indicate number of subjects; (S) indicates significant.
The level of significance for Chi-square test was taken as p<0.05.

Table 4.5.4 - Frequency of attending social gatherings by the women in the four BMI categories; n=387; % (n)						
Frequency	N (n=90)	PO (n=61)	OW (n=156)	Ob (n=80)	% Total (n=387)	P – value
Once a Week	11.4 (4)	0	57.1 (20)	31.4 (11)	9.0 (35)	<0.001 (S)
Twice a Month	0	30.4 (7)	26.1 (6)	43.5 (10)	5.9 (23)	
Once a month	25.0 (19)	0	39.5 (30)	35.5 (27)	20.0 (76)	
Occasionally	26.5 (67)	21.3 (54)	39.5 (100)	12.7 (32)	65.4 (253)	

Parentheses indicate number of subjects; (S) indicates significant.
The level of significance for Chi-square test was taken as $p<0.05$.

Table 4.5.5 - Pattern of eating in social gatherings by the women in the four BMI categories; n=387; % (n)						
Pattern of eating	N (n=90)	PO (n=61)	OW (n=156)	Ob (n=80)	% Total (n=387)	P – value
Full meals	44.4 (51)	16.5 (19)	39.1 (45)	0	29.7 (115)	0.001 (S)
Two items of a meal	100.0 (33)	0	0	0	8.5 (33)	-
Only snacks, beverages and desserts	3.3 (6)	19.0 (35)	47.8 (88)	29.9 (55)	47.6 (184)	<0.001 (S)
Only desserts	0	17.5 (7)	57.5 (23)	25.0 (10)	10.3 (40)	<0.001 (S)
Only beverages	0	0	0	100.0 (15)	3.9 (15)	-

Parentheses indicate number of subjects; (S) indicates significant.
The level of significance for Chi-square test was taken as $p<0.05$.

Table 4.6.1 - Nature of jobs of the women in the four BMI categories; n =185; % (n)						
Job type	N (n=40)	PO (n=23)	OW (n=80)	Ob (n=42)	% Total (n=185)	P – value
Desk job	12.0 (14)	7.7 (9)	51.3 (60)	29.1 (34)	63.2 (117)	<0.001 (S)
Touring/moving in office	50.0 (8)	43.8 (7)	0	6.2 (1)	8.7 (16)	
Standing	34.6 (18)	13.5 (7)	38.5 (20)	13.5 (7)	28.1 (52)	

Parentheses indicate number of subjects; (S) indicates significant.
The level of significance for Chi-square test was taken as $p<0.05$.

4.5.4 Frequency of attending social gatherings

Attending social gathering like marriage parties, birthday parties and other social functions is an important parameter for judging any person's frequency of eating out because socialising is always associated with food consumption. It was observed from table 4.5.4 that frequency of attending social gatherings once a week was significantly higher ($p<0.001$) for women in OW and Ob as compared to PO and N, but only 9.0% was the frequency in the sample.

4.5.5 Pattern of eating in social gatherings

The 387 women in the study were analysed for their preference of eating in social gatherings as shown in table 4.5.5. The data revealed that significantly higher ($p=0.001$) women in N preferred taking full meals or any two items of a meal as compared to the women in other three categories. On the other hand majority women in OW, Ob and PO preferred taking snacks, beverages and desserts.

4.6 ACTIVITY PATTERN

Activity pattern is an important indicator of one's lifestyle. Therefore, the daily activity pattern of the 387 subjects was analysed for type of job, time spent in various activities of daily routine along with time spent in sleeping, watching television and with children. The results of the activity pattern have been described in the following sections.

4.6.1 Nature of job

Nature of job had a significant influence on the weight status of women in the four BMI categories as observed in table 4.6.1. Out of the total 185 women working outside home, 63.2% were involved in desk jobs. In this group significantly higher ($p<0.001$) number of women were in OW (51.3%) as compared to 29.1% in Ob, just 12.0% and 7.7% in N and PO respectively. Thus significantly more number of women in OW and Ob had sedentary nature of job as compared to N and PO.

4.6.2 Domestic help

Household physical activity is an important parameter of energy expenditure. However, nowadays people are largely dependent upon domestic helps and labour saving devices. It results in saving physical effort and has a significant impact on the women's' weight status. This trend is largely prevalent in the high socio-economic status. Therefore, an insight into the kind of domestic helps employed by the study subjects will give a better understanding of their physical activity pattern. Table 4.6.2 revealed that 66.5% women in the study sample had a full time domestic help. Among these women, significantly higher ($p<0.001$) belonged to OW (47.6%) and Ob (23.2%) as compared to just 16.9% in N and 12.2% in PO. The within group analysis revealed that the use of part time domestic help was highest for N (52.2%) and least for OW (22.4%). Thus indicating that the use of part time domestic help increases physical activity and is a significant factor affecting weight status.

Table 4.6.2 - Type of domestic help employed by the women in the four BMI categories; n=387; % (n)

Type of help		N (n=90)	PO (n=61)	OW (n=156)	Ob (n=80)	% Total (n=387)	P – value
Part time	% in sample	35.3 (47)	22.6 (30)	26.3 (35)	15.8 (21)	34.4 (133)	<0.001 (S)
	% within group	52.2 (47)	49.2 (30)	22.4 (35)	26.3 (21)		
Full time	% in sample	16.9 (43)	12.2 (31)	47.6 (121)	23.2 (59)	65.6 (254)	
	% within group	47.8 (43)	50.8 (31)	77.6 (121)	73.8 (59)		

Parentheses indicate number of subjects; (S) indicates significant.
The level of significance for Chi-square test was taken as $p<0.05$.

4.6.3 Household activities

Women have to do various household activities, which require considerable physical effort. Therefore, in the present study the physical activity pattern of the subjects was studied with respect to the performance and non-performance of various household activities, frequency of performing these activities as well as the time spent in performing these activities.

4.6.3.1 Various household activities performed

The women were mostly performing activities like cooking, dusting, washing clothes, ironing, table laying and gardening. The results have been tabulated in table 4.6.3.1.

Table 4.6.3.1 - Percentage women performing various household activities in the four BMI categories; n=387; % (n)

Activity		N (n=90)	PO (n=61)	OW (n=156)	Ob (n=80)	% Total (n=387)	P – value
Cooking	% in sample	37.2 (61)	15.2 (25)	32.3 (53)	15.2 (25)	42.4 (164)	<0.001 (S)
	% within group	67.8 (61)	41.0 (25)	34.0 (53)	31.3 (25)		
Washing utensils	% in sample	0	0	0	0	0	-
	% within group	0	0	0	0		
Dusting	% in sample	35.1 (53)	17.2 (26)	31.8 (48)	15.9 (24)	39.0 (151)	<0.001 (S)
	% within group	58.9 (53)	42.6 (26)	30.8 (48)	30.0 (24)		
Sweeping	% in sample	0	0	0	0	0	-
	% within group	0	0	0	0		
Moping	% in sample	0	0	0	0	0	-
	% within group	0	0	0	0		
Washing Clothes	% in sample	40.7 (59)	13.1 (19)	28.3 (41)	17.9 (26)	37.5 (145)	<0.001 (S)
	% within group	65.6 (59)	31.2 (19)	26.3 (41)	32.5 (26)		
Ironing	% in sample	15.2 (17)	29.5 (33)	42.0 (47)	13.4 (15)	29.0 (112)	<0.001 (S)
	% within group	18.9 (17)	54.1 (33)	30.1 (47)	18.8 (15)		
Table laying	% in sample	32.7 (53)	16.7 (27)	38.9 (63)	11.7 (19)	41.9 (162)	<0.001 (S)
	% within group	58.9 (53)	44.3 (27)	40.4 (63)	23.8 (19)		
Watering plants	% in sample	20.4 (22)	18.5 (20)	50.0 (54)	11.1 (12)	27.9 (108)	0.009 (S)
	% within group	24.4 (22)	32.8 (20)	34.6 (54)	15.0 (12)		

Parentheses indicate number of subjects; (S) indicates significant.
The level of significance for Chi-square test was taken as $p<0.05$.

It was observed that significantly higher ($p<0.001$) number of women in N category were performing household activities like cooking, dusting and washing clothes in comparison to women in other three categories.

On the other hand, activities like ironing clothes, table laying and gardening were reported performed by significantly higher ($p<0.001$) number of women in OW as compared to N, PO and Ob. It was also observed that percentage women performing various household activities was significantly lower ($p<0.001$) for women in Ob among the four BMI categories. Also, none of the women in the four BMI categories were performing active physical household chores like washing clothes, sweeping and mopping.

Thus performance or non-performance and kind of household activities performed was a significant factor affecting the weight status of the women in the present study.

4.6.3.2 Frequency of performing various household activities

The data on frequency of performing various household activities has been given in table 4.6.3.2.

The frequency data revealed that significantly higher number of women belonging to N were performing household chores like cooking ($p=0.001$), dusting ($p=0.002$) and washing clothes ($p<0.001$) daily, as compared to women in PO, OW and Ob. However, significantly higher ($p<0.001$) women in OW and PO were performing the household activity of ironing clothes daily as compared to women in N and Ob. The frequency of watering plants as an activity was not significantly different ($p=0.086$) with respect to its performance for the women in the four categories.

Thus, the frequency of performing various household chores was significantly different among weight categories.

Table 4.6.3.2 - Frequency of performing various household activities by the women in the four BMI categories; n=387; % (n)

(a) COOKING (n=164)

Frequency	N (n=61)	PO (n=25)	OW (n=53)	Ob (n=25)	% Total (n=164)	P – value
Daily	44.5 (61)	14.6 (20)	29.2 (40)	11.7 (16)	83.5 (137)	0.001 (S)
Once a week	0	18.5 (5)	48.2 (13)	33.3 (9)	16.5 (27)	

(b) DUSTING (n=151)

Frequency	N (n=53)	PO (n=20)	OW (n=48)	Ob (n=24)	% Total (n=151)	P – value
Daily	44.0 (51)	14.7 (17)	25.0 (29)	16.4 (19)	76.8 (116)	0.002 (S)
Alternate day	0	50.0 (1)	50.0 (1)	0	1.3 (2)	
Twice a week	33.3 (1)	33.3 (1)	0	33.3 (1)	2.0 (3)	
Once a week	3.3 (1)	23.3 (7)	60.0 (18)	13.3 (4)	20.0 (30)	

(c) WASHING CLOTHES (n=145)

Frequency	N (n=59)	PO (n=19)	OW (n=41)	Ob (n=26)	% Total (n=145)	P – value
Daily	52.5 (42)	16.2 (13)	17.5 (14)	13.8 (11)	55.2 (80)	<0.001 (S)
Alternate day	53.8 (14)	7.7 (2)	23.1 (6)	15.4 (4)	17.9 (26)	
Twice a week	0	16.7 (2)	33.3 (4)	50.0 (6)	8.3 (12)	
Once a week	11.1 (3)	7.4 (2)	63.0 (17)	18.5 (5)	18.6 (27)	

(d) IRONING (n=112)

Frequency	N (n=17)	PO (n=33)	OW (n=47)	Ob (n=15)	% Total (n=112)	P – value
Daily	10.5 (11)	30.5 (32)	44.8 (47)	14.4 (15)	93.8 (105)	<0.001 (S)
Alternate day	100.0 (3)	0	0	0	2.7 (3)	
Once a week	75.0 (3)	25.0 (1)	0	0	3.6 (4)	

(e) WATERING PLANTS (n=108)

Frequency	N (n=22)	PO (n=20)	OW (n=54)	Ob (n=12)	% Total (n=108)	P – value
Daily	21.2 (11)	17.3 (9)	51.9 (27)	9.6 (5)	48.2 (52)	0.086 (NS)
Alternate day	38.5 (5)	0	61.5 (8)	0	12.0 (13)	
Once a week	14.0 (6)	25.6 (11)	44.2 (19)	16.3 (7)	39.8 (43)	

Parentheses indicate number of subjects; (S) indicates significant; (NS) indicates not significant. The level of significance for Chi-square test was taken as $p<0.05$.

4.6.3.3 Time spent in various household activities

Time spent in performing household activity is as important as the type and frequency of performing the activity. The mean time spent along with the standard deviation was calculated for various household activities with respect to the four BMI categories, the data for which has been given in table 4.6.3.3. On ANOVA, it was observed that significantly higher ($p<0.001$) mean time was spent in cooking by women in N as compared to the women in the other three categories. On the other hand mean time spent in dusting was significantly higher ($p=0.017$) for women in OW as compared to that for N, PO and Ob. But, as mentioned earlier that the frequency of performing dusting daily was significantly lower ($p=0.002$) for women in OW as compared to N.

Therefore, it can be said that since more number of OW women were performing the household chores of dusting once a week, so they spent greater time in it. It was also noted that the mean time spent in washing clothes was significantly higher ($p=0.016$) for women in OW and Ob as compared to N and PO.

However, within group analysis revealed that the difference between the mean time spent in washing by women in N & OW and N & Ob was not significant but was significant only with respect to PO.

The mean time spent in ironing was significantly higher ($p<0.001$) for women in N as compared to the other three categories. But the mean time spent in table laying was significantly higher ($p<0.001$) for women in OW and Ob in comparison to N and PO.

Also, the mean time spent in watering plants was significantly higher ($p=0.008$) for PO and Ob as compared to N and OW.

Thus, the time spent in performing various household chores was significantly different among different weight categories.

Table 4.6.3.3 - Mean time spent in various household activities by the women in four BMI categories; mean in minutes ± SD with range)						
Activity	N (n=90)	PO (n=61)	OW (n=156)	Ob (n=80)	Total (n=387)	P – value
Cooking	40.0 ± 24.23[a] (20-120)	30.0 ± 9.78[a1] (10-40)	20.0 ± 9.95 (10-60)	20.0 ± 8.29 (10-40)	28.0 ± 18.47 (10-120)	<0.001 (S)
Dusting	20.0 ± 8.8 (10-60)	22.5 ± 11.8 (10-60)	28.0 ± 16.3[b] (10-60)	20.6 ± 12.6 (10-60)	23.2 ± 12.8 (10-60)	0.017 (S)
Washing clothes	44.0 ± 27.69 (15-150)	25.0 ± 20.6[c] (10-90)	50.0 ± 29.5 (10-150)	55.0 ± 33.1 (15-120)	45.0 ± 29.24 (10-150)	0.016 (S)
Ironing	30.0 ± 18.09[d] (10-60)	15.0 ± 5.15 (10-30)	10.0 ± 4.9 (5-30)	15.0 ± 5.6 (10-30)	16.9 ± 9.7 (5-60)	<0.001 (S)
Table laying	9.0 ± 1.94[e] (5-10)	9.0 ± 1.98[e1] (5-10)	12.0 ± 2.3 (7-15)	11.0 ± 4.3 (5-15)	10.0 ± 2.6 (5-15)	<0.001 (S)
Watering plants	15.0 ± 7.02[f] (10-30)	25.0 ± 16.0 (10-60)	20.0 ± 12.3[f1] (10-60)	30,0 ± 18.3 (10-60)	20.0 ± 13.4 (10-60)	0.008 (S)

The level of significance for ANOVA was taken as p<0.05; (S) indicates significant.

Time spent in cooking; (ANOVA)
[a] - N > PO, OW, Ob   [a1] - PO > OW

Time spent in dusting; (ANOVA)
[b] - OW > N, Ob

Time spent in washing clothes; (ANOVA)
[c] - PO < N, OW, Ob

Time spent in ironing; (ANOVA)
[d] - N > PO, OW, Ob

Time spent in table laying; (ANOVA)
[e] - N < OW, Ob   [e1] - Po < OW, Ob

Time spent in gardening; (ANOVA)
[f] - N < PO, Ob   [f1] - OW < Ob

4.6.4 Travelling out for holiday

Travelling out for holiday is a stress buster but involves extra physical activity, which is important to evaluate while assessing the factors affecting the weight status. Therefore, in the present study frequency of holidaying and the activities of interest taken up during holidays were observed. The results are tabulated in tables 4.6.4.1 (a) and (b) and 4.6.4.2.

4.6.4.1 Frequency of holidaying

The data on frequency of holidaying has been given in Table 4.6.4.1. Almost 81.7% of sample were regularly holidaying. It was observed that significantly higher ($p<0.001$) women in Ob (92.5%) were regular travelers as compared to women in N, PO and OW.

Table 4.6.4.1 Frequency of travelling out for holiday by the women in the four BMI categories; n=387; % (n)

Frequency		N (n=90)	PO (n=61)	OW (n=156)	Ob (n=80)	Total (n=387)	P – value
Regularly	% in sample	24.1 (76)	12.7 (40)	39.9 (126)	23.4 (74)	81.7 (316)	<0.001 (S)
	% within group	84.4 (76)	65.6 (40)	80.8 (126)	92.5 (74)		
Occasionally	% in sample	19.7 (14)	29.6 (21)	42.3 (30)	8.5 (6)	18.3 (71)	
	% within group	15.6 (14)	34.4 (21)	19.2 (30)	7.5 (6)		

Parentheses indicate number of subjects; (S) indicates significant.
The level of significance for Chi-square test was taken as $p<0.05$.

4.6.4.2 Activities of interest during vacations

Preferred activities during vacations were sleeping/meditating, chatting, trekking, playing cards, leisure walks and sightseeing and spa treatment as depicted in table 4.6.4.2.

Table 4.6.4.2 - Preferred physical activities during vacations by the women in the four BMI categories; n=387; % (n)

Activity	N (n=90)	PO (n=61)	OW (n=156)	Ob (n=80)	% Total (n=387)	P – value
Trekking / Jogging	57.7 (30)	1.9 (1)	17.3 (9)	23.1 (12)	13.4 (52)	<0.001 (S)
Sleeping/Meditating	10.1 (20)	14.6 (29)	40.9 (81)	34.3 (68)	51.2 (198)	<0.001 (S)
Long distance walks	41.5 (68)	14.6 (28)	29.9 (49)	14.0 (23)	42.4 (164)	0.044 (S)
Sitting and chatting	15.4 (40)	20.1 (52)	39.4 (102)	25.1 (65)	66.9 (259)	<0.001 (S)
Playing cards	5.1 (9)	8.6 (15)	46.3 (81)	40.0 (70)	45.2 (175)	0.002 (S)
Sightseeing/spa	22.1 (59)	18.0 (48)	35.2 (94)	24.7 (66)	69.0 (267)	0.011 (S)

Parentheses indicate number of subjects; (S) indicates significant.
The level of significance for Chi-square test was taken as $p<0.05$.

The data revealed that significantly higher ($p<0.001$) number of women in OW (39.4%) preferred sitting and chatting with friends and family members during vacations as compared to 15.4% in N. Also, 42.4% women reported going out for leisure walks. Among these significantly higher ($p=0.044$) women were in N as compared to OW, PO and Ob. Going out of sight seeing or taking spa was reported by 69.0% women among which significantly higher ($p=0.011$) were in OW as compared to other three categories. As compared to N and PO, significantly higher ($p<0.001$) women in OW (40.9%) and Ob (34.9%) preferred sleeping/meditating when on holiday. Passive pass time activity like playing cards or board games were also significantly higher ($p=0.002$) for women in OW and Ob as compared to N and PO.

On the other hand active pursuits like trekking and jogging were significantly higher ($p<0.001$) for women in N as compared to the other three categories. Thus the kind of physical activity indulged in during vacations was a significant factor affecting the weight status of the women in the four BMI categories.

4.6.5 Preference for stairs/elevators/escalators

Cities are full of high rise buildings, whether it be residential or commercial building. Therefore, the people have to climb up and down. To ease moving up and down the high rise buildings the facility of elevators and escalators is generally provided along with the staircase. Use of stairs for climbing up and down leads to greater physical work as compared to the use of elevators/escalators. Therefore, in the present study, the preference of the subjects with respect to the use of stairs, elevators and escalators was analysed.

4.6.5.1 Preference while climbing up

Table 4.6.5.1 depicts the preference of the subjects for climbing up. It was observed that significantly higher ($p<0.001$) subjects in N preferred taking stairs while climbing up as compared to that in PO, OW and Ob.

Table 4.6.5.1 - Preference for stairs/elevators/escalators for climbing up by the women in the four BMI categories; n=387; % (n)

Preference		N (n=90)	PO (n=61)	OW (n=156)	Ob (n=80)	% Total (n=387)	P – value
Stairs	% in sample	49.2 (58)	19.5 (23)	23.7 (28)	7.6 (9)	30.5 (118)	<0.001 (S)
	% within group	64.4 (58)	37.7 (23)	17.9 (28)	11.3 (9)		
Escalators	% in sample	20.9 (18)	10.5 (9)	62.8 (54)	5.8 (5)	22.2 (86)	
	% within group	20.0 (18)	14.8 (9)	34.6 (54)	6.35 (5)		
Elevators	% in sample	7.7 (14)	15.8 (29)	40.3 (74)	36.1 (66)	47.3 (183)	
	% within group	15.6 (14)	47.5 (29)	47.4 (74)	82.5 (66)		

Parentheses indicate number of subjects; (S) indicates significant.
The level of significance for Chi-square test was taken as $p<0.05$.

Whereas, significantly higher ($p=0.011$) women in OW preferred escalators and elevators were preferred by significantly higher ($p<0.001$) women in Ob. Thus, the use of stairs, escalators and elevators was a significant factor affecting the weight status of women in the study.

4.6.5.2 Preference while climbing down

The preference for stairs/elevators/escalators while climbing down has been shown in table 4.6.5.2. It was observed that in comparison to 30.5% women preferring to take stairs while climbing up, 65.1% women reported taking stairs for climbing down. Among these, significantly higher ($p=0.01$) women belonged to OW and N as compared to PO and Ob. Again the preference for elevators was significantly higher ($p<0.001$) for women in OW, Ob and PO as compared to N. Thus, the preference for stairs and elevators was a significant factor affecting the weight status of the women.

4.6.6 Mode of commuting to places in the neighborhood

It is not the distance but the availability of time which governs our choice for commuting to places in the neighborhood like the local market, dropping children at the bus stop etc. In the present study, under the physical activity pattern, the women subjects were asked about the choice they make for commuting to places in the neighborhood. The results have been tabulated in the table 4.6.6.

Table 4.6.5.2 - Preference for stairs/elevators/escalators for climbing down by the women in the four BMI categories; n=387; % (n)

Preference		N (n=90)	PO (n=61)	OW (n=156)	Ob (n=80)	% Total (n=387)	P – value
Stairs	% in sample	31.7 (80)	15.5 (39)	39.7 (100)	13.1 (33)	65.1 (252)	0.01 (S)
	% within group	88.9 (80)	63.9 (39)	64.1 (100)	41.3 (33)		
Escalators	% in sample	11.4 (4)	25.7 (9)	48.6 (17)	14.3 (5)	9.0 (35)	0.186 (NS)
	% within group	4.4 (4)	14.8 (9)	10.9 (17)	1.3 (5)		
Elevators	% in sample	6.0 (6)	13.0 (13)	39.0 (39)	42.0 (42)	25.8 (100)	<0.001 (S)
	% within group	6.7 (6)	21.3 (13)	25.0 (39)	52.5 (42)		

Parentheses indicate number of subjects; (S) indicates significant.
The level of significance for Chi-square test was taken as $p<0.05$.

Table 4.6.6 - Preference of mode of commuting to neighbourhood places by the women in four BMI categories; n=387; % (n)

Mode	N (n=90)	PO (n=61)	OW (n=156)	Ob (n=80)	% Total (n=387)	P – value
By foot	24.6 (74)	15.9 (48)	39.2 (118)	20.3 (61)	78.0 (301)	0.160 (NS)
By transport	18.6 (16)	15.1 (13)	44.2 (38)	22.1 (19)	22.2 (86)	

Parentheses indicate number of subjects; (S) indicates significant.
The level of significance for Chi-square test was taken as $p<0.05$.

It was observed that 78.0% women preferred walking to nearby places, and just 22.0% used motorised transport. No significant difference (p=0.016) was observed among the four BMI categories with respect to the preference for mode of commuting to neighbourhood places.

4.6.7 Leisure time activities

The choice of activities preferred by people during their leisure time in the day can have a significant influence on their body weight status. In addition to this the length of sleeping time also has a significant impact on the weight status. Therefore, in the present study women were analyzed for their preference for various leisure time activities, and the time spend for sleeping, sitting, standing and walking.

4.6.7.1 Preference to do exercise during leisure time

Table 4.6.7.1 depicts the percentage women preferring exercise during leisure time. There was no significant difference (p=0.072) among the women in four BMI categories with respect to preference or non-preference for exercise during leisure time.

Table 4.6.7.1 - Preference to do exercise during leisure time by the women in four BMI categories; n=387; % (n)

Preference	N (n=90)	PO (n=61)	OW (n=156)	Ob (n=80)	% Total (n=387)	P – value
Exercise	17.7(34)	16.7(32)	42.2(81)	23.4(45)	192	0.072 (NS)
Do not exercise	28.7(56)	14.9(29)	38.5(75)	17.9(35)	195	

Parentheses indicate number of subjects; (NS) indicates not significant.
The level of significance for Chi-square test was taken as p<0.05.

4.6.7.2 Type of exercise or physical activity preferred during leisure

The data on preference for the type of exercise or physical activity indulged in by the women in their leisure time has been given in table 4.6.7.2. It was observed that 37.0% women preferred brisk walking. Among these, significantly higher (p<0.001) women were in OW (39.1%) and significantly lower were in PO (12.6%). Almost comparable percentage of women were in N and Ob. But, within group analysis revealed that significantly higher (p<0.001) women of Ob preferred brisk walking during leisure. Further, leisure walk as a pastime activity was more popular (42.1%) than brisk walking.

In this group, again significantly higher ($p=0.01$) women belong to OW (49.1%), but significantly lower were in Ob (6.1%).

The within group analysis however revealed that significantly higher ($p=0.01$) women of N were going for a stroll during leisure as compared to the women of PO, OW and Ob.

The data also revealed that significant ($p=0.001$) number of women also visited the gymnasium during their leisure. Among these, 50.0% each belonged to OW and Ob, but none were in N and PO. The within group analysis revealed that significantly higher ($p=0.001$) women of Ob were going to the gymnasium during their leisure time.

Table 4.6.7.2 - Type of exercise or physical activity preferred by women in the four BMI categories; n=387; % (n)

Preference		N (n=90)	PO (n=61)	OW (n=156)	Ob (n=80)	% Total (n=387)	P – value
Brisk walking	% in sample	23.8 (34)	12.6 (18)	39.1 (56)	24.5 (35)	37.0(143)	<0.001 (S)
	% within group	37.8 (34)	29.5 (18)	35.9 (56)	43.8 (35)		
Leisure walk	% in sample	34.4 (56)	10.4 (17)	49.1 (80)	6.1 (10)	42.1 (163)	0.010 (S)
	% within group	62.2 (56)	27.8 (17)	51.3 (80)	12.5 (10)		
Yoga	% in sample	18.8 (12)	12.5 (8)	42.2 (27)	26.6 (17)	16.5 (64)	0.448 (NS)
	% within group	13.3 (12)	13.1 (8)	17.3 (27)	21.3 (17)		
Gymnasium	% in sample	0	0	50.0 (9)	50.0 (9)	4.7 (18)	0.001 (S)
	% within group	0	0	5.8 (9)	11.3 (9)		

Parentheses indicate number of subjects; (S) indicates significant; (NS) indicates not significant. The level of significance for Chi-square test was taken as $p<0.05$.

4.6.7.3 Participating in ladies club/social organization

The data on participation in ladies club or in social organization by the women in the study has been given in Table 4.6.7.3. More than half, i.e 52.0% women reported being an active member of atleast one club or social organization. Among these, significantly higher ($p<0.001$) women belong to OW (53.7%) as compared to 22.9% in Ob, 15.4% in PO and just 8.0% in N. Thus active participation in ladies club was a significant factor affecting the weight status of women in the present study.

An interesting fact that came out was that not only more number of women belonging to OW and Ob categories were active in ladies club/social organization but they had joined more than one club/organization in comparison to the women belonging to the N category.

Table 4.6.7.3 - Percentage women attending ladies club/social organization during leisure in the four BMI categories; n=387; % (n)

Member	N (n=90)	PO (n=61)	OW (n=156)	Ob (n=80)	% Total (n=387)	P – value
Active Member	8.0 (16)	15.4 (31)	53.7 (108)	22.9 (46)	52.0 (201)	<0.001 (S)
Not a member	39.8 (74)	16.1 (30)	25.8 (48)	18.3 (34)	48.0 (186)	

Parentheses indicate number of subjects; (S) indicates significant;
The level of significance for Chi-square test was taken as $p<0.05$.

4.6.7.4 Time spent in viewing television

Television viewing is an important recreational activity which takes away considerable part of our leisure time. Since television viewing is total a sedentary activity, therefore the amount of time spent on it greatly influences the physical activity pattern. In the present study, the time spent for television viewing was analysed. The results have been tabulated in table 4.6.7.4.

It was observed that significantly higher ($p<0.001$) time was spent in television viewing by the women in PO, OW and Ob as compared to N. Time spent in television viewing was found to be positively and significantly ($r=+0.284$; $p<0.001$) correlated with BMI.

Thus clearly reflecting greater time spent in sedentary pursuits like television viewing is a significant factor affecting the weights status of the women in the present study.

Table 4.6.7.4 - Time spent on television viewing in minutes by the women in four BMI categories; (mean in minutes ± SD with range)

	N (n=90)	PO (n=61)	OW (n=156)	Ob (n=80)	% Total (n=387)	P – value
Mean television viewing time (in minutes)	55.0 ± 41.9^{a} (10-240)	70.0 ± 48.8^{a1} (15-240)	90.0 ± 52.6 (15-300)	95.0 ± 49.0 (30-300)	80.0 ± 51.2 (10-300)	<0.001 (S)

The level of significance for ANOVA was taken as $p<0.05$; (S) indicates significant.
Time spent on television viewing; (ANOVA)
[a] - N < PO, OW, Ob
[a1] - PO < OW, Ob

4.6.7.5 Time spent with children

Looking after children is a laborious task. All the women reported spending time with children. The time ranged from talking and listening to teenage children to playing indoor and outdoor games and helping with their schoolwork for younger children. However, when the women were asked to specify the kind of games they played with their children, it was observed that they were all playing some kind of indoor game like cards and board games.

Upto 29.0% women reported playing outdoor games like badminton, throw ball or just running after each other as shown in Table 4.6.7.5.1. Among these women, significantly higher ($p<0.001$) were in OW as compared to the other three categories. However, within group analysis revealed that significantly higher ($p<0.001$) number of N (37.8%) played outdoor games with their children as compared to just 28.8% of

Ob, 28.2% of OW and 18.0% of PO. Thus, the kind of play indulged in during leisure was a significant factor affecting the weight status of women in the present study.

Table 4.6.7.5.1 - Percentage women playing outdoor games with their children in the four BMI categories; n=387; % (n)

Type of play		N (n=90)	PO (n=61)	OW (n=156)	Ob (n=80)	% Total (n=387)	P – value
Out door	% in sample	30.4 (34)	9.8 (11)	39.3 (44)	20.5 (23)	29.0 (112)	<0.001 (S)
	% within group	37.8 (34)	18.0 (11)	28.2 (44)	28.8 (23)		

Parentheses indicate number of subjects; (S) indicates significant.
The level of significance for Chi-square test was taken as $p<0.05$.

There was a significant difference ($p<0.001$) when it came to the mean time spent with children, which has been shown in table 4.6.7.5.2. It was observed that women in N (4.4 hrs) were spending significantly longer ($p<0.001$) time with their children as compared to women in PO (2.6 hrs), OW (3.2 hrs) and Ob (2.8 hrs). Time spent in playing outdoor games with child was negatively and significantly ($r=-0.197$; $p<0.001$) correlated with BMI. Thus, the amount of time spent with children significantly affected the weight status of the women in the present study

Table 4.6.7.5.2 - Time spent with children in hours/d by the women in four BMI categories; (mean in hour ± SD with range)

	N (n=90)	PO (n=61)	OW (n=156)	Ob (n=80)	Total (n=387)	P – value
Mean time spent with children (hours/d)	4.4 ± 2.1[a] (1-9)	2.6 ± 1.5[a1] (1-6)	3.4 ± 2.2 (1-10)	2.8 ± 2.41[a2] (1-15)	3.4 ± 2.2 (1-15)	<0.001 (S)

The level of significance for ANOVA was taken as $p<0.05$; (S) indicates significant.
Time spent with children; (ANOVA)
[a] - N > PO, OW, Ob [a1] - PO < OW [a2] - Ob < OW

4.6.7.6 Time spent on three mandatory physical activities, i.e sitting, standing and walking

The data on time spent in sitting, standing and walking has been given in table 4.6.7.6. The data revealed that the mean sitting time for N was significantly lower ($p<0.001$) as compared to PO, OW and Ob, but OW and Ob were significantly more than PO. Whereas, the mean standing time was significantly higher ($p<0.001$) for N as compared to other three categories and PO was more than OW and Ob. But OW was less than Ob.

However, the four categories did not differ significantly ($p=0.280$) with respect to mean walking time. Nevertheless, the comparison of the mean time spent in walking revealed that the mean walking time for women belonging to N category was higher than the women belonging to the other overweight categories.

Time spending in sitting was positively and significantly ($r=+0.184$; $p<0.001$) correlated with BMI. Thus time spent in sitting and standing was a significant factor affecting the weight status of the women in the study.

Table 4.6.7.6 - Time spent (hrs) in sitting, standing and walking by the women in four BMI categories; (mean in hour ± SD with range)

Activity	N (n=90)	PO (n=61)	OW (n=156)	Ob (n=80)	Total (n=387)	P – value
Sitting	5.9 ± 1.6^{a} (1-10)	7.6 ± 1.3^{a1} (5-10)	8.7 ± 1.4 (5-12)	8.4 ± 1.6 (3-11)	7.8 ± 1.8 (1-12)	<0.001 (S)
Standing	6.9 ± 1.7^{b} (3-12)	6.4 ± 1.6^{b1} (3-9)	5.5 ± 1.6^{b2} (3-10)	6.0 ± 1.8 (1-12)	6.1 ± 1.8 (1-12)	<0.001 (S)
Walking	3.6 ± 0.9 (1-5)	2.1 ± 0.8 (1-4)	1.6 ± 0.5 (1-2)	1.2 ± 1.1 (1-2)	2.2 ± 0.8 (1-5)	0.280 (NS)

The level of significance for ANOVA was taken as $p<0.05$; (S) indicates significant; (NS) indicates not significant..

Time spent in sitting; (ANOVA)

[a] - N < PO, OW, Ob

[a1] - PO > N; OW, Ob > PO

Time spent in standing; (ANOVA)

[b] - N > PO, OW, Ob

[b1] - PO > OW

[b2] - OW < Ob

4.6.7.7 Time spent in sleeping

The data in table 4.6.7.7 revealed that there is a significant difference (p=0.007) between the duration of sleep of the women belonging to the four BMI categories. The mean time spent on sleeping by women in Ob was significantly higher (p=0.007) than that spent by women in N, PO and OW.

Sleep time was positively, but not significantly (r=+0.092; p=0.071) correlated with BMI.

Thus sleeping time is a significant factor affecting the weight status of the women in the study.

Table 4.6.7.7 - Mean time spent in sleeping in minutes by the women in four BMI categories; (mean in minutes ± SD with range)

	N (n=90)	PO (n=61)	OW (n=156)	Ob (n=80)	Total (n=387)	P – value
Mean time spent in sleeping (minutes)	389 ± 41. 3[a] (330-510)	396 ± 44.4[a1] (330-510)	401 ± 47.0[a2] (300-510)	413 ± 51.7 (300-570)	400 ± 46.9 (300-570)	0.007 (S)

The level of significance for ANOVA was taken as $p<0.05$; (S) indicates significant.
Time spent in sleeping; (ANOVA)
[a] - N < OW, Ob   [a1] - PO < Ob   [a2] - OW < Ob

4.7 ANTHROPOMETRIC INDICATORS

In the following sections anthropometric measures like weight, height, waist circumference, hip circumference, waist hip ratio (WHR) and waist stature ratio (WSR) was mapped for the sample comprising of 25-45 yrs affluent urban women.

In the present study the sample was categorized based on BMI (Table 4.7). The prevalence of obesity (Ob) in the sample was 20.7% (n=80), overweight (OW) was 40.3% (n=156), pre-overweight or at risk of overweight (PO) was 15.8% (n=61) and normal (N) was 23.3% (n=90)

Table 4.7 - BMI categorization of the women in the study sample; (n=387)		
BMI Categorization	(n)	(%)
Normal (N) (18.5 – 22.9 Kg/m^2)	90	23.3
Pre-Overweight (PO) (23 – 24.9 Kg/m^2)	61	15.8
Over weight (OW) (25 – 29.9 Kg/m^2)	156	40.3
Obese (Ob) (≥ 30.0 Kg/m^2)	80	20.7

4.7.1 Mean anthropometric measurements

The data on mean anthropometric measurements has been given in table 4.7.1. The data revealed that the mean weight of N was significantly lower ($p<0.001$) as compared to that of PO, OW and Ob. The difference in mean body weight of N versus PO, N versus OW and N versus Ob was 5.7 kg, 12.14 kg and 26.61 kg respectively.

The mean height of N and PO was significantly higher ($p=0.032$) than that of OW, but not that of Ob. The four BMI categories differed significantly ($p<0.001$) with respect to the mean waist circumference (WC), mean hip circumference (HC), and WC and HC of N was significantly lower than PO, OW and Ob (ANOVA).

On ANOVA, the mean WHR of only OW was significantly higher ($p<0.001$) than that of N, PO, Ob. The WSR was significantly lower than other three weight categories on ANOVA.

Thus anthropometric parameters like weight, height, WC, WHR and WSR were significantly different for the women in four BMI categories. The ANOVA analysis shows agreement in significant differences for weight, WC, HC and WSR but not for height and WHR.

Table 4.7.1 - Comparison of anthropometric indicators of women in the four BMI categories; (n=387) (mean ± SD with range)

Anthropometric Parameter	N (n=90) BMI = 18.5-22.9	PO (n=61) BMI = 23.0-24.9	OW (n=156) BMI = 25-29.9	Ob (n=80) BMI ≥ 30	Total (n=387)	P – value
Mean age	34.6 $\pm$ 5.27 (25-45)	37.2 $\pm$ 5.01 (27-45)	37.0 $\pm$ 5.16 (25-45)	37.4 $\pm$ 5.18 (25-45)	36.5 $\pm$ 5.26 (25-45)	0.001 (S)
Mean BMI (Kg/m^2)	21.5 ± 0.78 (19.2-22.9)	23.9 ± 0.52 (23.0-24.7)	27.1 ± 1.38 (25.0-29.9)	32.7 ± 2.4 (30.0-40.2)	26.5 ± 4.12 (19.2-40.2)	N/A
Mean weight (Kg)	52.9 ± 3.3^{a} (45.0-60.9)	58.7 ± 4. 4^{a1} (50.9-69.0)	65.1 ± 5.9^{a2} (51.3-77.5)	79.6 ± 7.9 (61.4 – 104.0)	64.3 ± 10.8 (45-104)	<0.001 (S)
Mean height (cm)	156.8 ± 3.95 (148.5-167.0)	156.5 ± 5.12 (145.0-168.0)	154.9 ± 5.17^{b} (140.0-165.6)	155.8 ± 6.78 (142.0-168.5)	155.8 ± 5.33 140.0-168.5)	0.032 (S)
Mean waist circumference (cm)	73.2 ± 3.6^{c} (61.0-80.0)	77.3 ± 3.9^{c1} (70.0-86.0)	83.5 ± 5.1^{c2} 72.0-97.0)	92.4 ± 7.9 74.0-113.0)	81.9 ± 8.6 (61.0-113.0)	<0.001 (S)
Mean hip circumference (cm)	90.9 ± 6.3^{d} (75.0-102.0)	95.6 ± 6.9^{d1} (80.0-110.0)	100.3 ± 6.2^{d2} 80.0-116.0)	115.3 ± 7.6 82.0-130.0)	100.5 ± 10.7 75.0-130.0)	<0.001 (S)
Mean waist hip ratio (WHR)	0.81 ± 0.05 (0.71-0.91)	0.81 ± 0.07 (0.65-0.91)	0.84 ± 0.06^{e} (0.72-0.97)	0.80 ± 0.08 (0.66-0.93)	0.82 ± 0.06 (o.65-0.97)	<0.001 (S)
Mean waist stature ratio (WSR)	0.38 ± 0.29^{f}	0.49 ± 0.03^{f-1}	0.54 ± 0.03^{f-2}	0.59 ± 0.06	0.53 ± 0.06	<0.001 (S)

The level of significance for ANOVA was taken as $p<0.05$; (S) indicates significant; (N/A) not applicable

Weight; (ANOVA)
^{a} - N < PO, OW, Ob; ^{a1} - PO < OW, Ob; ^{a2} - OW < Ob
Height; (ANOVA)
^{b} - OW < N, PO
Waist circumference; (ANOVA)
^{c} - N < PO, OW, Ob; ^{c1} - PO < OW, Ob; ^{c2} - OW < Ob
Hip circumference; (ANOVA)
^{d} - N < PO, OW, Ob; ^{d1} - PO < OW, Ob; ^{d2} - OW < Ob
WHR; (ANOVA)
^{e} - OW > N, PO, Ob
WSR; (ANOVA)
^{f} - N< PO, OW, Ob; $^{f-1}$ – PO < OW, Ob; $^{f-2}$ - OW < Ob

4.7.2 Abdominal Obesity

Abdominal obesity amongst the study population was evaluated with respect to waist circumference, WHR and WSR. The results have been tabulated in tables 4.7.2.1 (a) & (b), 4.7.2.2 and 4.7.2.3

4.7.2.1 Waist Circumference

The abdominal obesity data as observed from table 4.7.2.1(a) revealed that more than half, i.e 56.6% women had abdominal obesity on the basis of the cut-off value of < 80 cm of waist circumference for Asian women (WHO, 2004; Misra et al, 2005). In this group 53.0% women belonged to OW, 36.1% were Ob, 10.5% were PO and just 0.5% were N.

The four BMI categories differed significantly (p<0.001) with respect to the occurrence of abdominal obesity. Significantly, higher number of women in the OW and Ob categories had abdominal obesity as compared to women in the N and PO category.

Table 4.7.2.1 (a) - Occurrence of abdominal obesity in four BMI categories based on waist circumference criteria (WC<80.0cm); n=387; % (n)

Abdominal Obesity		N (n=90)	PO (n=61)	OW (n=156)	Ob (n=80)	% Total (n=387)	P – value
Waist Circumference (>80.0 cm)	% in sample	0.5 (1)	10.5 (23)	53.0 (116)	36.1 (79)	56.6 (219)	<0.001 (S)
	% within group	1.1 (1)	38.0 (23)	74.4 (116)	98.8 (79)		
Waist Circumference (<80.0 cm)	% in sample	53.0 (89)	22.6 (38)	23.8 (40)	0.6 (1)	43.4 (168)	
	% within group	98.9 (89)	62.3 (38)	25.6 (40)	1.3 (1)		

Parentheses indicate number of subjects; (S) indicates significant.
The level of significance for Chi-square test was taken as p<0.05.

Also, the within group analysis with respect to the occurrence of abdominal obesity revealed that 98.8% of obese women had abdominal obesity, as compared to 74.4% of OW, and just 38% of PO and only 1.1% of N.

Table 4.7.2.1(b) gives the distribution of subjects for abdominal obesity at action level-I for Asians. Action level-I by the group indicates first level prevention of metabolic syndrome by diet, exercise and weight management. The evaluation of subjects with waist circumference cut-off of ≥ 72.0 cm (action level-I for Asians,

Misra et al, 2006) revealed that 92.2% of women had waist circumference greater than or equal to 72.0 cm. Amongst these, 43.7% belonged to OW, 22.4% to Ob. However, upto 19.0% N and 15.1% PO had waist circumference at action level-I.

The within group analysis revealed that 74.4% of N, 88.5% of PO and 100.0% of OW and Ob women had waist circumference ≥ 72.0 cm. Thus indicating that women belonging not only to overweight and obese BMI category, but also the women belonging to normal and pre-overweight BMI category had waist circumference in the action level –I. There was a significant difference (p<0.001) between the four BMI categories with respect to occurrence of abdominal obesity at action level – I for Asians.

Table 4.7.2.1 (b) - Percentage of women in four BMI categories at action level – I of abdominal Obesity, waist circumference < 72.0 cm; n=387; % (n)

Abdominal Obesity		N (n=90)	PO (n=61)	OW (n=156)	Ob (n=80)	% Total (n=387)	P – value
Waist Circumference (≤ 71.9 cm)	% in sample	76.7 (23)	23.3 (7)	0	0	7.7 (30)	<0.001 (S)
	% within group	25.6 (23)	11.5 (7)	0	0		
Waist Circumference (≥ 72.0cm) (Action Level-I)	% in sample	18.8 (67)	15.1 (54)	43.7 (156)	22.4 (80)	92.3(357)	
	% within group	74.4 (67)	88.5 (54)	100.0 (156)	100.0 (80)		

Parentheses indicate number of subjects; (S) indicates significant.
The level of significance for Chi-square test was taken as p<0.05.

4.7.2.2. Waist to Hip Ratio (WHR)

Table 4.7.2.2 depicts the distribution of subjects on the basis of WHR criteria of occurrence of abdominal obesity at WHR > 0.85 for women (Hodge et al, 1993; Shetty, 2000). It was observed that the abdominal obesity amongst the study subjects came down to 31.0% when studied with respect to the WHR. In the group significantly higher (p<0.001) women were in OW (50.0%) as compared to just 21.7% in Ob, 17.5% in PO and 10.8% in N.

Table 4.7.2.2 - Occurrence of abdominal obesity in four BMI categories based on WHR (>0.85) n=387; % (n)							
Abdominal Obesity		N (n=90)	PO (n=61)	OW (n=156)	Ob (n=80)	% Total (n=387)	P – value
WHR > 0.85	% in sample	10.8 (13)	17.5 (21)	50.0 (60)	21.7 (26)	31.0 (120)	<0.001 (S)
	% within group	14.4 (13)	34.4 (21)	38.5 (60)	32.5 (26)		
WHR < 0.85	% in sample	28.8 (77)	15.0 (40)	36.0 (96)	20.2 (54)	69.0 (267)	
	% within group	85.6 (77)	65.6 (40)	61.5 (96)	67.5 (54)		

Parentheses indicate number of subjects; (S) indicates significant.
The level of significance for Chi-square test was taken as p<0.05.

4.7.2.3 Waist Stature Ratio (WSR)

The table 4.7.2.3 depicts abdominal obesity in subjects with respect to WSR. On the basis of WSR cutoff of ≥ 0.5 (Garnett et al, 2008; Ashwell and Hsieh, 2005), abdominal obesity was observed in 258 (66.7%) women, of which significantly higher (p<0.001) women belonged to OW (56.6%) as compared to 27.5% to Ob, 13.2% to PO and just 2.7% to N. However, the within group analysis revealed that significantly higher (p<0.001) women of OW (93.6%), Ob (88.8%) and PO (55.7%) as compared to those of N (7.8%) had abdominal obesity on the basis of WSR cutoff of ≥ 0.5.

Table 4.7.2.3 - Occurrence of abdominal obesity in four BMI categories on basis of waist-stature ratio (WSR ≥ 0.5); n=387; % (n)							
Abdominal Obesity		N (n=90)	PO (n=61)	OW (n=156)	Ob (n=80)	% Total (n=387)	P – value
(WSR ≥ 0.5)	% in sample	2.7 (7)	13.2 (34)	56.6 (146)	27.5 (71)	66.7 (258)	<0.001 (S)
	% within group	7.8 (7)	55.7 (34)	93.6 (146)	88.8 (71)		
(WSR < 0.5)	% in sample	64.3 (83)	20.9 (27)	7.8 (10)	7.0 (9)	33.3 (129)	
	% within group	92.2 (83)	44.3 (27)	6.4 (10)	11.2 (9)		

Parentheses indicate number of subjects; (S) indicates significant.
The level of significance for Chi-square test was taken as p<0.05.

Hence abdominal obesity in the sample was 56.6% according to waist circumference (> 80.0 cm); 92.3% according to waist circumference (≥ 72.0 cm); 31.0% according to WHR (> 0.85) and 66.7% according to WSR (≥ 0.5). The WHR criteria under reports the abdominal obesity as compared to WC and WSR.

4.8 BODY COMPOSITION

Body composition parameters like percent body fat (PBF), fat mass (FM), fat free mass (FFM), total body water (TBW), fat free mass index (FFMI) and fat mass index (FMI) were assessed on TANITA Body Composition Analyser TBF-300 for all 387 subjects during a health camp. The results have been tabulated in the sections below.

4.8.1 Mean Body Composition parameters

The mean of body composition parameters like percent body fat (PBF), fat mass (FM), fat free mass (FFM), total body water (TBW), fat free mass index (FFMI) and fat mass index (FMI) are depicted in table 4.8.1. It was observed that percent body fat of the subjects belonging to the four BMI categories consistently increased with the BMI category. The mean PBF was highest for the subjects belonging to the Ob category at 50.1% followed by the subjects belonging to OW at 41.3%. The PO category had mean PBF at 36.1%, which is > 35% while mean PBF of N was 30.5%. On ANOVA the PBF was significantly higher ($P<0.001$) for the subjects belonging to the three overweight categories as compared to the subjects belonging to the N category.

Like PBF, the mean fat mass (FM) of the subjects belonging to the three overweight BMI categories was significantly higher (ANOVA) than the mean fat mass of the subjects belonging to N. The mean FM of N category subjects was 16.2 kg, whereas it was 22.2 kg, 27.0 kg and 39.7 kg for the subjects belonging to PO, OW and Ob category respectively.

Fat free mass (FFM) was significantly different ($p=0.001$) for the four BMI categories. The mean FFM of the sample was 38.0 kg. It was 36.8 kg for subjects belonging to N, 37.5 kg for PO, 38.3 kg for OW and 39.4 kg for Ob BMI category.

However, the multiple-comparison test (post-hoc test) revealed that the mean FFM of the subjects belonging to N category was significantly lower (p=0.001) from the mean FFM of the subjects belonging to OW and Ob category. Even Ob was significantly higher (ANOVA) than OW and PO.

Table 4.8.1 - Comparison of body composition parameters of four BMI categories; (n=387) (mean ± SD with range)

Body composition	N (n=90)	PO (n=61)	OW (n=156)	Ob (n=80)	Total (n=387)	P – value
Mean PBF (%)	30.5 ± 3.2[a] (22.9-34.3)	36.1 ± 3.2[a1] (28.2-41.9)	41.3 ± 5.3[a2] (15.1-52.6)	50.1 ± 6.8 (40.3-64.3)	39.8 ± 8.3 (15.1-64.3)	<0.001 (S)
Mean FM (Kg)	16.2 ± 2.0[b] (10.8-20.3)	22.2 ± 8.2[b1] (16.9-81.9)	27.0 ± 4.5[b2] (9.7-36.2)	39.7 ± 7.4 (22.5-62.1)	26.3 ± 9.6 (9.7-81.9)	<0.001 (S)
Mean FFM (Kg)	36.8 ± 2.7[c] (31.5-42.6)	37.4 ± 3.4[c1] (31.4-49.2)	38.3 ± 4.7[c2] (29.8-54.2)	39.4 ± 6.1 (25.8-53.7)	38.0 ± 4.6 (25.8-54.2)	0.001 (S)
Mean TBW (Kg)	26.9 ± 1.9 (23.1-31.2)	27.4 ± 2.5 (23.0-36.0)	27.6 ± 3.9 (20.0-39.7)	28.9 ± 4.5[d] (18.9-39.3)	27.7 ± 3.6 (18.9-39.7)	0.003 (S)
Mean TBW (%)	50.8 ± 2.3[e] (40.2-56.4)	46.7 ± 2.2[e1] (42.5-52.8)	42.5 ± 4.8[e2] (30.9-62.1)	36.4 ± 5.0 (26.2-46.4)	43.8 ± 6.4 (26.2-62.1)	<0.001 (S)
Mean FFMI (Kg/m^2)	14.9 ± 0.7[f] (13.7-16.4)	15.3 ± 0.7[f1] (13.7-17.5)	15.9 ± 1.3 (13.7-21.4)	16.2 ± 2.1 (11.9-21.4)	15.6 ± 1.4 (11.9 – 21.4)	<0.001 (S)
Mean FMI (Kg/m^2)	6.5 ± 0.8[g] (4.6-7.7)	9.1 ± 3.4[g1] (6.9 – 34.9)	11.2 ± 1.8[g2] (3.8-15.6)	16.3 ± 3.0 (9.2-23.6)	10.8 ± 4.0 (3.8-34.9)	<0.001 (S)

The level of significance for ANOVA was taken as p<0.05; (S) indicates significant.

PBF; (ANOVA)
[a] - N < PO, OW, Ob; [a1] - PO < OW, Ob; [a2] - OW < Ob
FM; (ANOVA)
[b] - N < PO, OW, Ob; [b1] - PO < OW, Ob; [b2] - OW < Ob
FFM; (ANOVA)
[c] - N < OW, Ob; [c1] - PO < Ob; [c2] - OW < Ob
TBW; (ANOVA)
[d] - Ob > N, PO, OW
Percentage TBW (ANOVA)
[e] - N > PO, OW, Ob; [e1] - PO > OW, Ob; [e2] - OW > Ob.
FFMI; (ANOVA)
[f] - N < OW, Ob; [f1] - PO < OW, Ob.
FMI; (ANOVA)
[g] - N < PO, OW, Ob; [g1] - PO < OW, Ob; [g2] - OW < Ob

The mean total body water (TBW) (in Kg) of the subjects belonging to Ob category was highest at 28.9 Kg and significantly higher (ANOVA) than N, PO and OW. The mean TBW of the subjects belonging to N category was the least amongst the four BMI categories at 26.9 Kg as observed from Table 4.8.1. On the other hand, the mean percentage TBW of N was highest and significantly higher ($p<0.001$) than that of the other three categories. The mean percent TBW was inversely related to the BMI category. It was highest for N and least for Ob. The mean FFMI of the Ob and OW women were significantly higher ($p<0.001$) than that of N and PO. Also, the mean FMI of N was significantly lower ($p<0.001$) than that of PO, OW and Ob.

Thus, the body composition data indicates that all mean body composition parameters were significantly higher for women in OW and Ob as compared to N and PO.

4.8.2 Percent Body Fat (PBF)

In the present study, using the cutoff value of < 30.0%, the women were categorized on the basis of their PBF values as shown in table 4.8.2.

Table 4.8.2 - PBF cut-off used in the study to classify women in the four BMI categories

PBF range (%)	Significance
20.0 – 29.9	Acceptable
30.0 – 34.9	Overweight
≥ 35.0	Obesity

Source: Dudeja et al, 2001; Siddhu, 2004

The PBF value ≥ 30.0% and ≥ 35.0% was used to classify overweight and obesity in Indian women (Dudeja et al, 2001; Siddhu, 2004). The results have been tabulated in table 4.8.2.1. The analysis of PBF of 387 subjects revealed that only 9.0% (n=35) had the PBF value within the acceptable range of 20.0% – 29.9% as shown in Table 4.8.2.

In this group 82.9% were in N as compared to just 14.3% in OW and 2.9% in PO, and none off the Ob women were in this group. The within group analysis revealed that just 32.2% of N, 1.6% of PO and 3.2% of OW women had acceptable PBF values.

The data also revealed that 23.8% women in the sample had PBF value between 30.0% - 34.9%. This PBF range indicates overweight. Therefore, in the present study 23.8% women were overweight on the basis of the PBF criteria. Among these, significantly higher ($p<0.001$) women were in N (66.3%) as compared to PO (23.9%) and OW (9.8%). However, none among these belong to Ob. It was observed that when this data was analysed within group, 67.8% women of N had excess fat as compared to 36.1% of PO and 5.8% of OW. Thus indicating that significant number of women with normal BMI were over fat (> 30% PBF) in the study.

The PBF value ≥ 35.0% was considered as obesity. On this basis 67.2% of the study sample was obese. In this group, significantly higher ($p<0.001$) number of women belonged to OW (54.6%) as compared to Ob (30.8%) and PO (14.6%) and none belonged to N. However, within group analysis revealed that all the 80 obese women were obese by the PBF cutoff criteria also. Upto 91.0% of OW and 62.3% of PO women were over fat > 35%. Thus indicating the high level of obesity in the study subjects on the basis of PBF cutoff.

Table 4.8.2.1 - Distribution of Subjects on basis of Percent Body Fat (PBF) cutoff of < 30.0%; n=387; % (n)

PBF Range (%)		N (n=90)	PO (n=61)	OW (n=156)	Ob (n=80)	% Total (n=387)	P value
20.0 - 29.9	% in sample	82.9 (29)	2.9 (1)	14.3 (5)	0	9.0 (35)	<0.001 (S)
	% within group	32.2 (29)	1.6 (1)	3.2 (5)	0		
30.0 – 34.9	% in sample	66.3 (61)	23.9 (22)	9.8 (9)	0	23.8 (92)	
	% within group	67.8 (61)	36.1 (22)	5.8 (9)	0		
≥ 35.0	% in sample	0	14.6 (38)	54.6 (142)	30.8 (80)	67.2 (260)	
	% within group	0	62.3 (38)	91.0 (142)	100.0 (80)		

Parentheses indicate number of subjects; (S) indicates significant.
The level of significance for Chi-square test was taken as $p<0.05$.

4.9 DIETARY INTAKE

The dietary intake of the 387 subjects was evaluated for energy, protein, fat intake and intake of other nutrients. All the nutrient intakes were compared with the respective recommended dietary allowance of ICMR (2010) as well as ICMR (1990). The mean intake with the range and ANOVA has been given in the table 4.9.

Energy - The mean energy intake was highest for the subjects belonging to OW category at 1998 Kcal/d and lowest for N (1634 Kcal/d) among the four BMI categories as observed from table 4.9. This value was 5.26% (+99 Kcal) more than the raised energy intake value of 1899 Kcal/d for sedentary Indian women in ICMR (2010). On the other hand, the gap between recommended and actual intake of N was 14.0% (-265 Kcal/d). The mean intake of Ob (1690 Kcal/d) was comparable to that of N and was 11.0% (-2.9 Kcal) less than the RDA (ICMR, 2010). This reflects that the women in the Ob category are either eating less in order to reduce weight or under reporting. On ANOVA, mean energy intake of OW was significantly higher ($p<0.001$) than that of N, PO and Ob. Also, N is significantly lower (ANOVA) than PO and OW but not Ob.

Protein - Like the mean energy intake, the mean protein intake was highest for the subjects belonging to OW category at 57.8 g and was closely followed by the subjects belonging to PO category with the mean intake of 57.4 g/d. The mean protein intake of the Ob category was lowest amongst the four BMI categories at 53.7 g/d, and was 2.4% (-1.3 g) less than the RDA (ICMR, 2010). There was no significant difference between the recommended (ICMR, 2010) and mean protein intake. But when compared with ICMR (1990) recommended protein intake of 50 g/d, the mean intake of all the categories was significantly higher ($P=0.014$).

The mean protein intake of Ob was significantly lower (ANOVA) than that of PO and OW, but was not significantly different from that of N.

Fat - The mean intake of fat (visible and invisible) per day for all the four categories was significantly higher ($p<0.001$) than the recommended (ICMR, 2010) intake of 30 g/d (both visible and invisible). The trend of consuming the most was maintained by the OW category at 67.5 g/d. The mean fat intake of subjects belonging to PO category was 64.8 g; and the mean fat intake of N and Ob category was same at 58.1g/d.

Also, the mean fat intake was significantly higher ($p<0.001$) for PO and OW as compared to N and Ob.

Carbohydrate - The mean carbohydrate intake of OW was highest at 289.5 g/d amongst the four BMI categories. This intake was significantly higher ($P<0.001$) than the mean carbohydrate intake of the other three BMI categories.

Calcium - There was no significant difference ($p=0.119$) between the mean calcium intake of the four BMI categories, but calcium intake was highest for Ob (960 mg) and least for N and OW (871 mg). However, when compared to the RDA value of 600 mg/d (ICMR, 2010) and value of 400 mg/d (ICMR, 1990), all the four categories were significantly higher than ($p<0.001$) the optimal value.

Iron - The mean dietary intake of iron (15.0 mg/d) was significantly lower ($p<0.001$) than new reduced allowance of 21.0 mg/d (ICMR, 2010). Amongst the four BMI categories, the highest mean iron intake was that of 15.9 mg/d of the subjects belonging to OW category. The mean iron intake of OW category was significantly higher ($p<0.001$) than that of other three categories, but there was no significant difference between the other three categories.

Vitamin A - Vitamin A consumption was studied in the form of retinol and beta-carotene. The mean intake of retinol was significantly lower ($p=0.003$) than the RDA of 600 μg/d (ICMR, 2010; ICMR 1990). Retinol intake was highest for N (530 μg/d) and lowest for Ob (348 μg/d). On the other hand, the intake of vitamin A in form of beta-carotene was highest for the subjects belonging to the Ob category at 7519.6 μg/d and lowest for N at 2621 μg/d. When compared to the recommended beta-carotene intake of 4800 μg/d in the ICMR (2010), the mean intake of subjects in the three categories i.e N, PO and OW, was significant lower but intake of Ob was significantly higher ($p<0.001$).

Table 4.9 - Nutrient intake of the women in the four BMI categories; (n=387) (mean ± SD with range)

Nutrient	RDA (ICMR, 1990)	RDA (ICMR, 2010)	N (n=90)	PO (n=61)	OW (n=156)	Ob (n=80)	Total (n=387)	P – value
Energy (Kcal)	1875	1899	1634 ± 234[a] (1151-2844)	1876 ± 266[a1] (1380-2645)	1998 ± 198[a2] (1580-2399)	1690 ± 378 (978-2844)	1830 ± 306 (978-2844)	<0.001 (S)
Protein (g)	50	55	56.1 ± 8.1 (39.5-82.3)	57.4 ± 9.1 (40.0-88.5)	57.8 ± 8.5 (42.0-72.7)	53.7 ± 12.9[b] (30.8-88.8)	56.5 ± 9.7 (30.8-88.8)	0.014 (S)
Fat (g)	-	-	58.1 ± 12.7[c] (37.5-88.8)	64.8 ± 13.3[c1] (40.5-97.3)	67.5 ± 13.3[c2] (44.8-93.0)	58.1 ± 17.4 (32.2-95.1)	62.9 ± 14.7 (32.2-97.3)	<0.001 (S)
Carbohydrate (g)	-	-	229 ± 49[d] (137-423)	260 ± 62[d1] (137-391)	289 ± 42[d2] (236-408)	229 ± 53 (134-423)	258 ± 56 (134-423)	<0.001 (S)
Calcium (mg)	400	600	871 ± 370 (400-1594)	931 ± 320 (407-1594)	871 ± 269 (457-1690)	960 ± 269 (321-1495)	899 ± 305 (321-1690)	0.119 (NS)
Iron (mg)	30.0	21.0	14.1 ± 2.6 (8.2-18.3)	14.6 ± 3.0 (9.4-22.2)	15.9 ± 3.5[e] (9.6-23.8)	14.7 ± 4.2 (8.2-24.6)	15.0 ± 3.5 (8.2-24.6)	<0.001 (S)
Retinol (µg)	600	600	530 ± 227 (201-1435)	501 ± 312 (170-1603)	465 ± 416.8 (169-1608)	348 ± 243.4[f] (112-1440)	462 ± 336.1 (112-1608)	0.003 (S)
Beta Carotene (µg)	2400	4800	2621 ± 1437[g] (190-9100)	3929 ± 5034[g1] (190-36000)	4752 ± 3951 (590-14885)	7519 ± 4901 (190-16588)	4691 ± 4279 (190-36000)	<0.001 (S)
Vitamin-C (mg)	40	50	84.6 ± 49.6[h] (40-257)	121.1 ± 61.5[h1] (45-62)	137.3 ± 44.1 (83-225)	133.8 ± 57.4 (52-257)	121.7 ± 55.3 (40-262)	<0.001 (S)
Thiamine (mg)	1.1	1.0	1.25 ± 0.37[i] (0.57-2.16)	1.43 ± 0.38 (0.57-2.57)	1.51 ± 0.4 (1.1-2.4)	1.77 ± 2.6 (0.68-2.5)	1.49 ± 1.25 (0.57-2.57)	0.054 (S)
Riboflavin (mg)	1.3	1.1	1.44 ± 0.28 (1.1–2.1)	1.4 ± 0,29 (0.8-2.3)	1.31 ± 0.26 (0.8-1.9)	1.6 ± 0.92[j] (0.6-3.5)	1.44 ± 1.7 (0.6-3.5)	0.053 (S)

However, in comparison to the 1990 recommended allowance of 2400 μg/d, the intake of PO, OW and Ob was significantly higher and that of N was comparable to the recommended intake.

Vitamin– C - The mean intake of vitamin-C was highest for OW (133.8 mg/d) and lowest for N (84.6 mg/d). When compared with the recommended intake of 50 mg/d (ICMR, 2010). The mean intake of all the four categories was significantly higher ($p<0.001$). Amongst the four categories, the mean intake of vitamin-C was significantly lower (ANOVA) for N as compared to PO, OW, Ob. Also, on ANOVA PO was significantly lower ($p<0.001$) than OW and Ob.

Thiamin and Riboflavin – The mean intake of thiamin and riboflavin was significantly higher ($p=0.003$) than the RDA (ICMR, 2010) and ICMR (1990). Intake of Thiamin was significantly lower ($p=0.054$) for N as compared to that of Ob. However, it was not significantly different for PO and OW. Intake of riboflavin was significantly higher ($p=0.05$) for Ob as compared to the other three categories.

The level of significance for ANOVA was taken as $p<0.05$; (S) indicates significant. (ANOVA for Table 4.9)

Energy Intake; (ANOVA)
[a] - N < PO, OW; [a1] - PO < OW; PO > Ob [a2] - OW > Ob

Protein Intake; (ANOVA)
[b] - Ob < PO, OW

Fat Intake; (ANOVA)
[c] - N < PO, OW; [c1] - PO > Ob; [c2] - OW > Ob

Carbohydrate Intake; (ANOVA)
[d] - N < PO, OW; [d1] - PO < OW; PO > Ob [d2] - OW > Ob

Iron Intake; (ANOVA)
[e] - OW > N, PO, Ob

Retinol Intake; (ANOVA)
[f] - Ob < N, PO, OW

Beta-Carotene Intake; (ANOVA)
[g] - N < PO, OW, Ob; [g1] - PO < Ob [g2] - OW < Ob

Vitamin-C Intake; (ANOVA)
[h] - N < PO, OW, Ob; [h1] - PO < OW

Thiamine Intake; (ANOVA)
[i] - N < Ob

Riboflavin Intake; (ANOVA)
[j] - Ob > N, PO, OW

4.9.1 Relative contribution of three proximate principles in total day's energy intake (TDEI)

The analysis of meal composition of the four BMI categories as depicted in table 4.9.1 revealed that the carbohydrate is the chief contributor of the calories in the diet of the women in the study. Carbohydrate energy percent of OW was significantly higher (p=0.026) than that of PO and Ob, but it was comparable to that of N. However, the protein energy percent of N was significantly higher (P<0.001) than that of the other three categories. Even that contribution of fat energy was significantly higher (p=0.042) for N as compared to that of OW and Ob.

Table 4.9.1 - Total day's energy Intake (TDEI) and relative contribution of proximate principles in the four BMI categories; (n=387) (mean ± SD with range)

Parameters	N (n=90)	PO (n=61)	OW (n=156)	Ob (n=80)	Total (n=387)	P – value
TDEI (Kcal)	1634 ± 234^{a} (1151-2844)	1876 ± 266^{a1} (1380-2645)	1998 ± 198^{a2} (1580-2399)	1690 ± 378 (978-2844)	1830 ± 306 (978-2844)	<0.001 (S)
Carbohydrate En%	56.1 ± 8.9 (39.4-77.3)	55.5 ± 9.4^{b} (24.0-71.7)	57.9 ± 5.1^{b1} (50.1-78.7)	55.1 ± 8.5 (24.0-77.1)	56.5 ± 7.7 (24.0-78.7)	0.026 (S)
Protein En %	13.8 ± 1.3^{c} (11.5-17.2)	12.3 ± 1.8^{c1} (8.8-17.2)	11.6 ± 1.2^{c2} (9.7-14.5)	12.8 ± 1.5 (8.1-15.8)	12.4 ± 1.7 (8.1-17.20	<0.001 (S)
Fat En %	32.1 ± 5.7^{d} (20.4-47.6)	31.2 ± 5.2 (18.1-43.5)	30.1 ± 4.4 (18.6-38.5)	30.6 ± 4.7 (22.9-44.2)	30.9 ± 4.3 (18.6-47.6)	0.042 (S)

The level of significance for ANOVA was taken as p<0.05; (S) indicates significant.

TDEI; (ANOVA)
^{a} - N < PO, OW, Ob; ^{a1} - PO < OW; PO > Ob; ^{a2} - OW > Ob

Carbohydrate En %; (ANOVA)
^{b} - PO < OW; ^{b1} - OW > Ob

Protein En %; (ANOVA)
^{c} - N > PO, OW, Ob; ^{c1} - PO > Ob; ^{c2} - OW < Ob

Fat En %; (ANOVA)
^{d} - N > OW, Ob

4.10 ENERGY EXPENDITURE AND ENERGY STATUS

The energy expenditure for the 387 subjects was studied with respect to the four BMI categories. Total day's energy expenditure (TEE) was estimated as well as the activity pattern of the subjects in the four BMI categories was evaluated.
Also, the mean TEE was compared with total day's energy intake (TDEI) to calculate the energy balance. The results have been tabulated in the following sections.

4.10.1 Total Energy Expenditure (TEE)

The mean TEE was estimated using the factorial technique, based on energy cost of activities given in FAO/WHO/UNU (2004). The results have been tabulated in tables 4.10.1.

The mean TEE of Ob was significantly higher ($p<0.001$) than that of N, PO and OW. TEE was lowest for PO at 2000 ± 117.9 Kcal per day and highest for Ob at 2243 ± 176.1 Kcal per day. However, TEE of N and OW were comparable.

Total energy expenditure (TEE) is influenced by basal metabolic rate (BMR) and physical activity level (PAL). The analysis of BMR and PAL data in table 4.10.1 revealed that the mean BMR of Ob was significantly higher ($p<0.001$) than that of the other three categories.

BMR of Ob was highest at 1452 ± 73.1 Kcal per day and was lowest for N at 1224 ± 34.9 Kcal per day.

On the other hand, the mean PAL was significantly higher for women in N as compared to the mean PAL of women in the other three categories. The mean PAL value was 1.69 for N and was 1.57, 1.56 and 1.55 respectively for Po, OW and Ob.

Table 4.10.1 - Mean total day's energy expenditure (TEE); total days' energy intake and other relative indices with respect to the four BMI categories; (n=387) (mean ± SD with range)

Parameters	N (n=90)	PO (n=61)	OW (n=156)	Ob (n=80)	Total (n=387)	P – value
Mean BMI (Kg/m^2)	21.5 ± 0.78 (19.2-22.9)	23.9 ± 0.52 (23.0-24.7)	27.1 ± 1.38 (25.0-29.9)	32.7 ± 2.4 (30.0-40.2)	26.5 ± 4.12 (19.2-40.2)	NA
Mean BMR Kcal/d)	1224 ± 34.9[a] (1076-1309)	1278 ± 44.3[a1] (1210-1432)	1327 ± 56.4[a2] (1120-1462)	1452 ± 73.1 (1297-1735)	1321 ± 94.9 (1076-1735)	<0.001 (S)
Mean TDEI (Kcal/d)	1634 ± 234 (1151-2844)	1876 ± 266 (1380-2645)	1998 ± 198[b] (1580-2399)	1690 ± 378 (978-2844)	1830 ± 306 (978-2844)	<0.001 (S)
Mean TEE (Kcal/d)	2079 ± 125.6[c] (1768-2490)	2000 ± 117.9[c1] (1749-2234)	2069 ± 145.2[c2] (1681-2660)	2243 ± 176.1 (1849-2671)	2096 ± 164.1 (1681-2671)	<0.001 (S)
Mean PAL	1.69 ± 0.08[d] (1.44-1.93)	1.57 ± 0.07 (1.38-1.70)	1.56 ± 0.08 (1.40-1.90)	1.55 ± 0.10 (1.36-1.82)	1.58 ± 0.11 (1.36-1.93)	<0.001 (S)

The level of significance for ANOVA was taken as p<0.05; (S) indicates significant; (NA) is not applicable

BMR; (ANOVA)
[a] - N < PO, OW, Ob; [a1] - PO < OW, Ob [a2] - OW < Ob

TDEI; (ANOVA)
[b] - OW > N, PO, Ob

TEE; (ANOVA)
[c] - N > PO; N < Ob [c1] - PO < OW, Ob [c2] - OW < Ob

PAL; (ANOVA)
[d] - N > PO, OW, Ob

4.10.2 Physical activity level (PAL) of the study subjects

FAO/WHO/UNU (2004) has recommended a PAL value of 1.75 to prevent obesity. Keeping this value as a cutoff, the women in the study sample were categorised. The results have been given in table 4.10.2. The data revealed that just 6.2% of the women had a PAL value ≥ 1.75. Amongst these 19 subjects 79.2% were in N, whereas, the remaining 93.8% of the study population were below this PAL value. Thus indicating that majority of the women were leading a sedentary life and were susceptible to weight gain. However, within group data revealed that significantly higher ($p<0.001$) percentage of N (21.1%) were moderately active i.e PAL ≥ 1.75 as compared to just 1.9% of OW, 2.5% of Ob and none of PO.

Table 4.10.2 - Percentage women with PAL value above or equal to 1.75 and below 1.75 in the four BMI categories; n=387; % (n)

PAL value		N (n=90)	PO (n=61)	OW (n=156)	Ob (n=80)	Total (n=387)	P – value
< 1.75	% in sample	19.6 (71)	16.8 (61)	42.1 (153)	21.5 (78)	93.8 (363)	<0.001 (S)
	% within group	78.9 (71)	100.0 (61)	98.1 (153)	97.5 (78)		
≥ 1.75	% in sample	79.2 (19)	0	12.5 (3)	8.3 (2)	6.2 (24)	
	% within group	21.1 (19)	0	1.9 (3)	2.5 (2)		

Parentheses indicate number of subjects; (S) indicates significant.
The level of significance for Chi-square test was taken as $p<0.05$.

4.10.3 Deriving cutoff of PAL for maintaining normo-weight in urban affluent women in the reproductive age group

FAO/WHO/UNU (2004) recommends a PAL value of 1.75 to prevent obesity. However, in the present study a mean PAL of 1.69 was obtained for the women belonging to N category whereas the mean PAL of OW and Ob was 1.56 and 1.55 respectively. In order to identify an appropriate cutoff value of PAL to maintain normal weight, receiver operating characteristic (ROC) curve was drawn when BMI ≤ 22.9 Kg/m^2 was taken as the standard (Fig. 4.10.3). It was observed that a PAL value of 1.64 gave the best sensitivity (82.22%) and specificity (83.84%) when area under the curve (AUC) was 0.861. The detail of this ROC curve analysis is given in **Annexure – 16**. The PAL value of 1.64 was much lower than FAO/WHO/UNU (2004) cutoff of 1.75. The FAO/WHO/UNU criteria of PAL > 1.75 to prevent obesity was desired because research data supports this value by the fact that weight regain was least in subjects with PAL > 1.7. This PAL value corresponds to moderate intensity activity of approximately 45 to 60 min/d (Schoeller et al, 1997; Weinsier et al, 2002; Saris et al, 2003). However, PAL value > 1.64 in the present study, is the activity level, which ensures BMI = 22.9 Kg/m^2 among N. Among affluent Indian women, who are growing to be more sedentary, ensuring a PAL of > 1.64 is fairly well associated with normal weight.

Fig. No. 4.10.3
(ROC curve to determine the appropriate value of PAL form BMI among affluent Indian women)

Surrogate BMI ≤ 22.9 Kg/m^2; AUC = 0.861

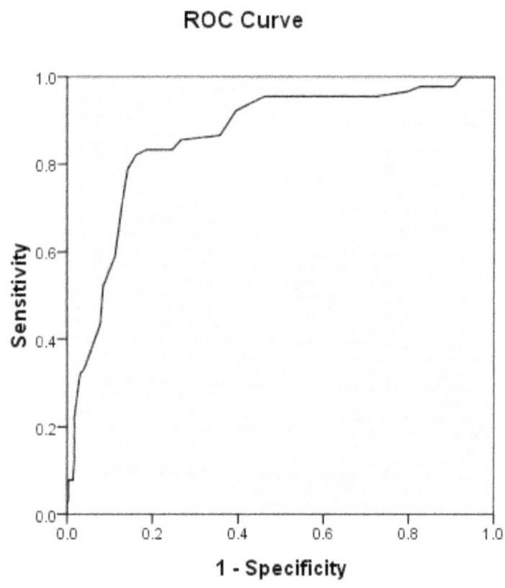

Diagonal segments are produced by ties.

4.10.4 Time Spent in Five Activity Categories

The total day's time of 24 hours was categorised into five activity categories suggested by FAO/WHO/UNU (2004) for each subject in the four BMI categories. The mean time spent along with the range in the five activities categories by the subjects in the four BMI categories has been tabulated in table 4.10.4.

It was observed that the mean time spent in sleep was significantly lower (p<0.001) for N in comparison to that spent by women in PO, OW and Ob. There was no significant difference between the mean sleeping time of the three overweight BMI categories amongst themselves when two categories were taken at a time.

There was no significant difference (p=0.342) in the mean time spent in obligatory activities by the women in the four BMI categories. The mean time spent in discretionary activities without exercise, which included general household work and leisure time activities was significantly higher (p<0.001) for women in N as compared to PO, OW and Ob.

The mean time spent in residual activities, like lying, personal care etc was significantly higher (p=0.004) for women in N and PO as compared to OW. However there was no significant difference with respect to the mean time spent in residual activities between OW and Ob and N, PO and Ob.

The mean time spent in exercise was significantly higher (p=0.002) for N as compared to other three categories.

Table 4.10.4 - Comparison of mean time spent in five activity categories in minutes in a day by the women in the four BMI categories; (n=387) (mean ± SD with range)

Activity	N (n=90)	PO (n=61)	OW (n=156)	Ob (n=80)	Total (n=387)	P – value
Sleep (min)	412.3 ± 61.2[a] (300-600)	460.3 ± 69.2 (360-600)	453.0 ± 83.2 (300-600)	447.0 ± 99.7 (300-600)	443.5 ± 82.1 (300-600)	<0.001 (S)
Obligatory (min)	428.7 ± 158.3 (120-720)	419.5 ± 211.1 (90-780)	463.2 ± 186.9 (120-780)	441.1 ±193.2 (180-780)	443.8 ± 186.2 (90-780)	0.342 (NS)
Discretionary without exercise (min)	354.3 ± 92.9[b] (120–480)	310.2 ± 134.6 (60-720)	307.0 ± 107.6 (60-540)	323.8 ± 86.4 (160-540)	322.0 ± 106.5 (60-720)	0.007 (S)
Residual (min)	217.8 ± 55.8[c] (120-360)	232.1 ± 75.5[c1] (120-390)	196.1 ± 67.5 (60-390)	210.1 ± 77.8 (100-390)	209.7 ± 69.6 (60-390)	0.004 (S)
Exercise (min)	30.4 ± 26.9[d] (0-90)	20.5 ± 27.2 (0-75)	21.1 ± 21.6 (0-60)	17.6 ± 21.3 (0-75)	22.5 ± 23.1 (0-90)	0.002 (S)

The level of significance for ANOVA was taken as p<0.05; (S) indicates significant; (NS) indicates not signigicant.

Sleep; (ANOVA)
[a] - N < PO, OW, Ob

Discretionary; (ANOVA)
[b] - N > PO, OW, Ob

Residual; (ANOVA)
[c] - N > OW [c1] - PO > OW

Exercise; (ANOVA)
[d] - N > PO, OW, Ob

4.10.5 Energy Status

The energy status of the study sample was calculated by subtracting the total energy expenditure of each subject from the total energy intake of that subject. The results have been tabulated in table 4.10.5 (a).

Although, only 23.5% (n=91) women in the study were in the positive balance but among these significantly higher ($p<0.001$) number of women belonged to OW (69.2%; n=63) as compared to 22.0% (n=20) in PO, 6.6% (n=6) in Ob and just 2.2% (n=2) in N.

Table 4.10.5 (a) - Percentage women in positive and negative energy balance in the four BMI categories; n=387; % (n)

Energy Status	N (n=90)	PO (n=61)	OW (n=156)	Ob (n=80)	% Total (n=387)	P – value
Positive Balance	2.2 (2)	22.0 (20)	69.2 (63)	6.6 (6)	23.5 (91)	<0.001 (S)
Negative Balance	29.6 (87)	13.9 (41)	31.3 (92)	25.2 (74)	76.0 (294)	
In balance	50.0 (1)	0	50.0 (1)	0	0.5 (2)	

Parentheses indicate number of subjects; (S) indicates significant. Balance = TEE - TDEI
The level of significance for Chi-square test was taken as $p<0.05$.

The mean energy balance of the women in the four categories as depicted in table 4.10.5 (b) revealed that although all the four categories were in negative balance, but the imbalance was highest for Ob (-562 Kcal) and lowest for OW (-71 Kcal). On ANOVA, energy imbalance of Ob was significantly higher ($p<0.001$) that PO and OW, but was not significantly different from that of N.

Table 4.10.5 (b) - Mean energy balance of the women in the four BMI categories; (n=387) (mean ± SD with range)

	N (n=90)	PO (n=61)	OW (n=156)	Ob (n=80)	Total (n=387)	P – value
Mean energy balance	-484 ±26.9[a] (-1006-603)	-156 ± 307.5[a1] (-803-605)	-71.1 ±252.5[a2] (-1074-516)	-562 ± 391.7 (-1265-460)	-282 ±367.6 (-1265-605)	<0.001 (S)

The level of significance for ANOVA was taken as $p<0.05$; (S) indicates significant.

Energy Balance; (ANOVA)
[a] - N > PO, OW ; [a1] - PO < N, Ob ; [a2] - OW < N, Ob ; [a3] - Ob > PO, OW

4.11 DETERMINANTS OF DESIRABLE BODY WEIGHT STATUS IN WOMEN

The univariate analysis (chi-square) of the various factors revealed that as many of 40 factors were determining the desirable body weight status of women in N category. The factors have been enlisted in table 4.11.1.

Table 4.11.1 Factors associated with desirable weights status of subjects in the four BMI categories

Sr. No.	Factor	P-value
1.	Younger age	0.001
2.	Less number of parity	0.001
3.	Nuclear family	0.002
4.	Lower family history of obesity, hypertension, heart disease and diabetes	0.001
5.	Normal weight status of parents	<0.001
6.	Higher age of onset of menarche	<0.001
7.	Higher age of marriage	0.001
8.	Higher age of parity	<0.001
9.	Not using oral contraceptive	0.004
10.	Post partum weight gain in the range of 3-4 Kg	<0.001
11.	Self perceived normal weight status	<0.001
12.	Mean weight gain and loss in the range of 2-3 Kg per annum	<0.001
13.	Ovo vegetarian diet	0.001
14.	Regular consumption of 3 main meals in a day	0.001
15.	Fixed eating amount	0.001
16.	Medium pace of eating	<0.001
17.	Eat preferably at fixed meal time	<0.001
18.	Eating normal meal once on a fasting day	<0.001
19.	Balance diet during pregnancy and lactation	<0.001
20.	Less fluctuation dietary behavior	<0.001

21.	Smart food choices when eating at home and outside	<0.001
22.	Lesser frequency of eating out	<0.001
23.	Less dependence on full time domestic help	<0.001
24.	Lower mean sitting time	<0.001
25.	Higher mean standing time	<0.001
26.	Greater participation in household activities	<0.001
27.	Higher frequency of performing household activities	<0.001
28.	Greater indulgence in higher energy expenditure activities while on holiday	0.001
29.	Greater preference for stairs even when there is a choice	<0.001
30.	Lower mean sleeping time	0.007
31.	Lower television viewing time	<0.001
32.	More time spent with children	<0.001
33.	More time spent in exercise	0.002
34.	PAL value of 1.69	<0.001

Along with the significant factors of desirable body weight status in women, certain significant outcomes of overweight/obese status were also observed which are shown in table 4.11.2.

Table 4.11.2 Outcome of overweight / obese weight status of women in the study		
Sr. No.	Outcome	p-value
1.	Irregular menstruation	0.022
2.	Difficulty in breast feeding	0.004
3.	Greater health monitoring	<0.001
4.	Higher morbidity	0.001
5.	Greater indulgence in adopting various weight reducing techniques	<0.001
6.	Change in past dietary behavior	<0.001

The multi-variate binary logistic regression analysis of the significant factors gave the final determinants of desirable body weight status of women in the present study. The determining factors have been given in table 4.11.3.

Table 4.11.3 Final determining factors affecting desirable body weight status of women of 25-45 years; (n=387)

Sr. No.	Determining factor	p-value	Odds ratio
1.	Family history of obesity, hypertension and heart disease.	<0.001	6.43
2.	Weight status of father	0.006	3.44
3.	Self perceived weight status	<0.001	57.026
4.	Tendency to overeat when hungry	<0.001	17.55
5.	Longer sitting time	<0.001	2.473
6.	Longer television viewing	0.001	1.013

1. In the present study family history of obesity, hypertension and heart disease came out as a significant factor ($p<0.001$) affecting the desirable body weight status of women. The binary logistic regression analysis revealed that the chance of occurrence of obesity in women is 6.43 times more with family history of obesity, hypertension and heart disease, in comparison to those who do not have the family history of these degenerative non-communicable diseases.

2. Weight status of father came out as a significant factor ($p=0.006$) affecting the weight status. It was observed that the chance of overweight/obesity is 3.4 times higher in women whose father is overweight or obese as compared to women whose father had normal weight.

3. In the present study self perceived weight status of women was a significant factor ($p<0.001$) affecting the desirable body weight status. The binary regression analysis revealed that correct perception of normal weight status

helps in maintaining normal body weight. It was observed that women correctly perceiving their body weight status as normal have a 57 times higher chance of being normal weight as compared to those women who perceived themselves as overweight.

4. Tendency to overeat when hungry was a significant factor ($p<0.001$) for overweight/obese status of women in the study. Statistical analysis reveal that women who tend to overeat have a 17.5 times greater chance of being overweight or obese as compared to women who have a fixed or regulated appetite.

5. Longer sitting time also came out as a significant factor ($p<0.001$) affecting weight status of women in the study. It was observed that women who sat for longer duration had 2.5 times greater chance of being overweight /obese as compared to women who sat for a shorter duration.

6. Longer television viewing time was also significantly ($p<0.001$) affecting the desirable body weight status of women. Binary logistic regression analysis revealed that women who viewed television for longer duration had 1.013 times greater chance of being overweight /obese as compared to women who watched television for a shorter duration.

The last two factors pertain to sedentary lifestyle and have emerged as important factors in all ages. FAO/WHO/UNO (2004) recommends moderate activity lifestyle insuring PAL > 1.75. Table 4.11.1 highlights association of sedentary lifestyle to weight status and significant contribution of exercise, less seated activity like watching television and high PAL in maintaining normo-weight status (PAL=1.69). Among host of other factors in Table 4.11.1, family history and father's weight status emerged to play significant role. The last significant determining factor was sensitivity to self image. It is quite possible that tracking one's own self image flags sequel of behaviour changes which ensure normo weight status.

Risk factors of metabolic syndrome among Asian Indians were studied by Ravikiran et al (2010) in 2225 subjects, ≥ 20 yrs of age living in Chandigarh, a city in North India. Like the present study, the risk factors for metabolic syndrome were identified through multiple logistic regression analysis, and they were found to be age, female gender, sedentary lifestyle and diabetes in parents. Looking at these risk factors and those identified in the present study (table 4.11.3) for overweight status, it can be commented that sedentary lifestyle, female gender and family history of NCD are the factors, which need to be highlighted in the community for both prevention and occurrence of disease.

4.11.4 Self attributed reasons for present weight status

The women were asked to list out the reasons for their present weight status. The reasons have been enlisted in table 4.11.4.

The women in the four categories gave various reasons for weight gain as well as for maintaining normal weight. It was observed that 54.8% women in the study group reported genetic reasons for their present weight status. Among these, significantly higher ($p<0.001$) were OW as compared to the other three categories. However, the within group analysis revealed that significantly higher ($p<0.001$) Ob women believed that their present overweight status is largely due to genetics. But, when other reasons were analyzed with respect to within group, it was observed that apart from genetics, significantly higher ($p<0.001$) women in OW and Ob were not only more sedentary, but also had an erratic lifestyle, which included frequent partying, poor self control, binge eating, skipping meals etc.

On the other hand, significantly higher ($p<0.001$) women in N category were conscious eaters and were leading an active life, which was a blend of exercise as well as regulated eating. Thus, clearly indicating that it was not only the genetic makeup that made the difference, but also the difference in the lifestyle, which set the two groups apart.

Also, it was observed that significantly higher percentage of OW and Ob women reported weight gain due to pregnancy, use of oral contraceptives, pregnancy related complications and weight cycles. However, none of the women in N had these problems. These points were further looked at through FGD in the following section i.e section 4.12.

Table 4.11.4 - Reasons attributed for present weight status by the women in the four BMI categories; n=387; % (n)

Reasons		N (n=90)	PO (n=61)	OW (n=156)	Ob (n=80)	% Total (n=387)	P – value
Genetics	% in sample	19.8 (42)	11.8 (25)	43.4 (92)	25.0 (53)	54.8 (212)	<0.001 (S)
	% with in group	46.7 (42)	41.0 (25)	59.0 (92)	66.3 (53)		
Conscious eating	% in sample	87.6 (78)	4.5 (4)	7.9 (7)	0	23.0 (89)	<0.001 (S)
	% with in group	86.7 (78)	6.6 (4)	4.5 (7)	0		
Stress	% in sample	12.1 (8)	13.6 (9)	33.3 (22)	40.9 (27)	17.1 (66)	<0.001 (S)
	% with in group	8.9 (8)	14.8 (9)	14.1 (22)	33.8 (27)		
Regular exercise and diet	% in sample	76.7 (46)	8.3 (5)	15.0 (9)	0	15.5 (60)	<0.001 (S)
	% with in group	51.1 (46)	8.2 (5)	5.8 (9)	0		
Erratic lifestyle	% in sample	0	7.3 (11)	59.3 (89)	33.3 (50)	38.8 (150)	<0.001 (S)
	% with in group	0	18.0 (11)	57.1 (89)	62.5 (50)		
Sedentary lifestyle	% in sample	0	7.3 (10)	59.1 (81)	33.6 (46)	35.4 (137)	<0.001 (S)
	% with in group	0	16.4 (10)	51.9 (81)	57.5 (46)		
Post pregnancy	% in sample	0	11.4 (15)	52.3 (69)	36.4 (48)	34.1 (132)	<0.001 (S)
	% with in group	0	24.6 (15)	44.2 (69)	60.0 (48)		
Use of oral contraceptives	% in sample	0	5.8 (4)	39.1 (27)	55.1 (38)	17.8 (69)	<0.001 (S)
	% with in group	0	6.6 (4)	17.3 (27)	47.5 (38)		
Abortions / miscarriage	% in sample	0	15.7 (11)	37.1 (26)	47.1 (33)	18.1 (70)	<0.001 (S)
	% with in group	0	18.0 (11)	16.7 (26)	41.3 (33)		
Weight cycle	% in sample	0	0	37.5 (21)	62.5 (35)	14.5 (56)	<0.001 (S)
	% with in group	0	0	13.5 (21)	43.6 (35)		

Parentheses indicate number of subjects; (S) indicates significant.
The level of significance for Chi-square test was taken as $p<0.05$.

4.12 FOCUS GROUP DISCUSSION

Issues surrounding weight are sensitive topics that elicit a complex set of attitudes and beliefs based on individual experiences and cultural practices. Therefore, a qualitative method involving discussion in a focus group setting allows obtaining perspectives about obesity and obesity management, without limiting participants to respond to a set of predetermined questions in a questionnaire. The use of focus group discussion technique helped to explore, in depth, this socially and personally sensitive subject. It also helped to gain insight into the factors perceived as barriers for weight reduction or maintenance after weight loss. Useful information was gathered from successful weight losers who have been able to maintain weight despite similar barriers.

In the present study risk factor mapping of factors effecting desirable weight status was done with the help of focus group discussion. The aim was to congregate participants in a non threatening location with an atmosphere that would encourage interactive and dynamic dialogue and sharing of views, ideas, experiences and feelings.

For the present study, five FGD's were conducted in five different localities in Delhi, namely

(i) C – Block South Extension, Part -2, New Delhi;
(ii) UNESCO Apartments, Patparganj, New Delhi;
(iii) Printers Apartments, Rohini, Delhi;
(iv) IB Block, Ashok Vihar, Phase-I, Delhi; and
(v) Surya Cooperative Society, Dwarka, New Delhi.

Women drawn from all walks of life, including professional working women, non-professional working women and mothers who were homemakers with desirable body weight and overweight in the age group of 25 to 50 years participated in focus group discussion (FGD). In each of the five discussions 8 to 10 women participated, a number considered optimal for effective focus group communication (Millward, 1995). The women were provided with information about the date and time of their focus group discussion. The location for the discussion was a community facility in the locality or the Housing Complex. Although, it was indicated that the discussion would be for 90 minutes approximately, but in most of the cases, the discussion extended upto two hours; because body weight is one subject, which interests all women irrespective of age and weight status. Tea and light snacks were served to the participants after the discussion.

The sample for FGD was contacted through Residential Welfare Association (RWA). The telephone numbers were obtained through the RWA,s directory available at the Residential Welfare Office. During the telephonic conversation information regarding socio-demographic and health related information, including age, weight and height was obtained. For use during the sessions, a list of open ended questions was developed to gather specific information and facilitate discussions concerning weight management and factors contributing to its success or failure. The theme questions are as follows:

(i) Is your body weight a cause of concern?
(ii) What reasons would you give for your present body weight status?
(iii) What methods you have adopted to lose/maintain your body weight?
(iv) Which methods worked best?
(v) Which methods did not show the results?
(vi) What is the contribution of your family members in your pursuit for desirable body weight?
(vii) What is the role of your neighborhood in maintaining weight?
(viii) How do you like to spend your leisure time?
(ix) Why is it difficult to lose weight?
(x) What is one burning comment or piece of information that you want to add, which I missed out?

The FGDs were conducted by a moderator and a notes taker, who had been trained to conduct the FGD in a standardized way.

The women were seated in a semi-circle with the moderator in the centre. The FGDs were conducted in Hindi and English. The discussions were audio-taped, with the consent of the participants. One sample of transcribed FGD has been given in **Annexure – 17.**

Analysis of the responses

The recorded discussions were transcribed by the moderator on the same day after the discussion using the notes taken by the observer to supplement the tape recordings. The Hindi scripts were translated verbatim into English by the moderator. The reports were interpreted on the basis of the theme questions. The findings with relevant discussion are presented in the succeeding paragraphs.

Findings and Discussion

(i) Concept of Overweight

The self perception of weight is a judgmental issue, which varies from women to women. Some overweight women considered themselves as normal because they were not suffering from any medical problem and are physically active.

> *"मैं तो मांनती हूँ की मैं normal हूँ, क्योंकि मुझे कोई medical problem नही है, और मैं अपना सारा काम फुर्ती से कर लेती हूँ, जबकि मुज़से पतले दिखने वाले कितने slow और सुस्त हैं".*

- Overweight woman of 35 years

While some normal weight women were concerned about their weight status

> *"मेरा weight आधा किलो भी बढ़जाता है तो मैं रोटी और चावल खाना छोड़ देती हूँ और सिर्फ़ salad और vegetables खाती हूँ"*

- Normal weight women of 30 years

Fittings of certain type of clothes also determined their perception of weight status.

"सलवार कुर्ते में तो मैं normal लगती हूँ पर jeans और t-shirt में मोटी लगती हूँ"

- Slightly overweight women of 29 years

Some women felt that being overweight makes them looks older than their age.

"A little weight gain is natural after marriage and child birth, but I have started looking overage and feel insecure about it."

- Overweight women of 32 years

The above findings show that although the self image of overweight varied from women to women, but most of them were more concerned about the cosmetic effect of weight gain.

(ii) Reasons for present weight status

The reasons given for present weight status varied from genes, post pregnancy weight gain, love for sweets and snacks, frequent partying, weight cycling, physical inactivity and menopause by overweight women. Genes, regularity in lifestyle, conscious eating were the three main factors quoted by most women with desirable bodyweight.

Most of the overweight women said that their inability to control their habit of overeating their favourite food, which in most of the cases was sweets and snacks, has led to weight gain.

"I do not eat much all the time but yes good food tempts me and I tend to overeat"

- Overweight women of 35 years

"Normally, I am conscious, but while talking on the phone or while watching television, I have this fascination of eating and land up finishing the entire packet of biscuits or chips"

- Overweight women of 36 years

"मैं kitchen में काम करते करते छे-सात biscuit ऐसे ही खा लेती हूँ"

- Overweight women of 34 years

On the other hand most of the women with desirable body weight felt that they were conscious while eating any kind of food, which included even their favorite food.

"I eat everything in routine. I neither under-eat nor overeat. I have a fixed appetite"

- Normal weight women of 35 years

"Thanks to my genes because I do not exercise at all. I only take care that I do not overeat at any point. I am basically a conscious eater. I eat everything but nothing in excess, so I think my weight is maintained."

- Normal weight woman of 38 years

Overweight women felt that their genetic makeup coupled with sedentary lifestyle led to their present weight status. Most of them could not lose the weight gained during pregnancy.

"I think it is in my family, my mother gained weight after me and my brother were born and same has been my case. I have gained a lot after my second child and have been gaining since then"

- Overweight woman of 38 years

"I have gained after childbirth because I did not bother for myself. No exercise and no fixed eating time"

- Overweight woman of 33 years

A few overweight women also felt that they gained weight when stressed because they had no other reason for weight gain.

"I start eating more when I am disturbed or worried"

- Overweight woman of 40 years

4. RESULTS

Most of the women in the age group 43-45 years felt that they suddenly become lethargic and feel tired by daily routine chores as a result do not have the energy/interest to indulge in any kind of physical activity. They blame this to the approaching menopause.

> *"मैं आजकल tired feel करती हूँ और weight भी जयादा हो गया है. मुझे लगता है की मेरी menopause की stage आ रही है क्योकि मैं 40+ तो हूँ ही"*

- Overweight woman of 43 years

But a few women in the same age group felt that these symptoms of menopause can be overshadowed if a regular exercise and eating routine is maintained over a life span.

> *"I am 45 years old and look I can put any 30 years old girl to shame because I am regular with my daily walk, which I have been doing for last 25 years. I have a fixed routine of eating, which I rarely change."*

- Normal weight women of 34 years

Also the habit of eating leftover food either from child's plate or consuming previous day's leftover food in small quantity, which otherwise cannot be served; was given as one of the reasons for weight gain.

> *"I was never the type to overeat but after marriage and childbirth, my mother-in-law strictly told me that child's leftover mild and food should be consumed and not wasted."*

- Overweight woman of 29 years

> *"I am like a dustbin of my house. I put all the previous day's leftover food in my stomach, since there are no takers for it."*

- Overweight woman of 38 years

However, some overweight women were unable to reason out for their excess weight despite being cautious about it.

"मैं ज़यादा खाती भी नही और थोड़ी बहुत exercise भी करती हूँ, पर फिर भी वज़न बढ़ जाता है"

- Overweight woman of 38 years

"I have a strange body. When I exercise daily by going to the gymnasium, I am able to lose weight, but the moment I give a break to this routine, the lost weight comes back."

- Overweight woman of 37 years

(iii) Techniques adopted to maintain / lose weight

The discussion revealed that most of the women with desirable body weight had been able to keep excess weight at bay because they had been able to work out right combination of physical activity with regulated eating in their life. These women also described specific personal strategies employed by them to maintain weight.

"I do brisk walking for 15 minutes every day in the morning while dropping my children at the bus stop"

- Normal weight women of 33 years

"I wear my jogging shoes the moment I get up so that I do not lie down *again"*

- Normal weight woman of 40 years

"I keep practicing pranayam while sitting in my office"

- Normal weight woman of 37 years

"I have started getting up 15 minutes early than my usual routine and take five rounds of the lane outside my house before starting with daily routine".

This participant reported that though she has not lost much weight, but she has not gained since then and feels more light and comfortable now.

- Overweight woman of 40 years

"मैं week में एक बार jeans और t-shirt ज़रूर पहनती हूँ, इससे मुझको weight का idea हो जाता है. Waist में थोड़ा सा फ़र्क भी पता चलता है जोकि सलवार और कमीज़ पहने पर नही पता चलता. इसलिये में ज़रूरी steps जैसे की diet पर control और walking करके weight वापिस अपने normal level पर ले आती हूँ."

- Slightly overweight woman of 35 years

"हमारे घर में बहुत ज़यादा party culture है पर में अपने साथ बहुत strict हूँ एक snack लेती हूँ और उसको ले कर धीरे धीरे खाती हूँ, ताकि जब तक सब लोग snack खा रहे हों तो मेरे हाथ में भी खाने की चीज़ हे. इससे किसी को पता भी नही लगता और मैं over eating नही कर पाती."

- Normal weight woman of 34 years

Similarly, another normal weight participant informed that she does not finish her glass of carbonated drink till the end of party so that she does not have to go for a re-fill. Also, she asserts to be very cautious in eating snacks, and never lets her plate of snacks get empty which naturally limits her snack intake. To maintain this she says that she slows her eating speed and takes very small morsels at a time. In this way, she avoids overeating snacks and drinking excessive cold drinks, without getting noticed.

"Since the time I was detected with borderline diabetes, I have stopped eating in parties and marriages. Before going out I take my meal, so that I do not feel hungry. Also, I have started walking in the evening. I

have been able to lose almost 7-8 kilograms in last 3 months. I feel more happy now."

- Now an overweight, but earlier obese women of 37 year

"Earlier I used to sit while my son was playing in the park with his friends. But now I also wear my shoes and walk for atleast half and hour in the walking track built along the park."

- Normal weight women of 38 years

It was also observed that overweight women had greater ideas regarding weight loss techniques and had made number of attempts at weight losing. The techniques employed by them varied from dieting, fasting, wearing fitted cloths, working out in gymnasium, going to a health clinic, spa, massage, ayurveda, naturo-pathy and practicing yoga or other physical activities.

"मुझ से dieting जितनी मर्ज़ी करवा लो पर में exercise नही कर सकती"

- 30 years old overweight woman

"I fast a lot"

- 40 years old slightly overweight woman

"I like wearing fitted clothes so I am aware of even a slight gain and quickly take the necessary action"

- 31 years old Normal weight woman

"I drink two glasses of hot water in the morning"

- 31 years old overweight woman

"I do treadmill for thirty minutes everyday in the gymnasium with my friends"

- 33 years old normal weight women

"I have enrolled for Shikha Sharms's weight loss program"

- 29 years old overweight women

"A Yoga instructor comes to our home every alternate day in the morning and make me and my husband do various exercises"

- 36 years old overweight woman

"I have started walking and avoiding fried foods and sweets because my cholesterol level has crossed the normal range and the doctor has warned me that if I do not lose weight, I should be prepared for a serious heart problem, which I do not want"

- 43 years old overweight women

Although most of the overweight women practicing various weight reduction techniques were still overweight but it was very clear that they had not passively accepted the incremental weight gain. They are continuously striving for the healthy size.

(iv) Techniques which worked and those which did not

Most of the women indicated that they were successful in losing weight but failed to maintain the weight loss. Like, women who had joined the gymnasium told that they gained weight moment they stopped going to the gymnasium. Also women who were following a dieting regime confessed that they could not carry on with that regime forever. Even the women who had gone for ayurveda and Naturopathy treatments reported that they got back to their original size after the program or the course was over.

"मैं जब तक health clinic में जाती रही मेरा weight कम रहा, पर जैसे ही मेरा program ख़तम हुआ और मैं वापिस अपने routine में आई तो जो weight loss किया था वो तो वापिस आया ही पर साथ extra weight भी gain किया"

- 34 years old overweight woman

On the other hand, women with healthy body size felt that conscious eating along with regular physical activity like walking, breathing exercises or yoga even for a short while like 15 minutes a day helps in maintaining weight status. These women felt that overweight women should not look for immediate weight loss because this kind of routine will help them achieve that but if this routine is followed on regular basis it will show results in the long run.

"Even I had put on lot of weight after my 2nd child and tried every possible way to lose but failed in all. Then I decided to do things my way. I am getting up just 15 minutes earlier than my regular schedule in order to do Pranayam. This has helped me in toning my body. In the afternoon, instead of talking on the telephone, I take a nap for 30 minutes. Earlier I used to watch T.V. at night, but now I try to sleep early so that I can get up on time. Now my situation is such that if I do not do my morning exercise, I feel uncomfortable throughout the day"

- 38 years old normal weight woman

Most of the women who participated in the FGD felt that techniques like practicing yoga/pranayam at home or walking for some time were the kind of physical activities which can be followed successfully in routine along with household responsibilities. On the other hand, techniques, which require longer time period or certain changes in their daily routine are more likely to fail because women perform multiple roles which at time do not blend with their aim of weight reduction.

(v) Role of family, friends and neighborhood

Most of the women felt that family, children, good locality, ability to wear the desired variety of clothing, improved social acceptance due to better physical appearance are the biggest motivators or enhancers of weight reduction and maintenance.

"My husband and children especially my daughter just don't let me gain weight. They start pointing moment I put on a little weight"

- 36 year old normal women

"My daughter does not let me make nor eat any fried product"

- *40 years old normal weight woman*

"My mother-in-law is so particular about her fitness that even I have become conscious because she looks so young"

- 38 years old overweight woman

"In our society we have a well built walking tracks and can walk at any point in time in the day"

- 35 years old normal weight woman

"We have formed a morning walking group. After dropping children at the bus stop we all walk for 15 minutes in the complex and whoever misses has to pay fine of Rs.500/- per day"

- 38 years old overweight women

"Earlier nobody commented on my appearance but after losing 10 kilograms, my friend and even my husband has started complimenting me and it is a real pleasure to hear good things about oneself"

- 33 years old slightly overweight woman

(vi) Leisure time activity

Leisure time for homemakers was the afternoon time, generally after lunch, when children either sleep or watch television; whereas working women reported that they hardly have any leisure time on the working days. Most of the women were either taking a nap, watching television, reading newspaper, talking on the telephone during their leisure time.

Leisure time for most women whether on a weekday or holiday ranged from 30-60 minutes.

"I have a fixed routine. I watch my favourite show from 3.00-3.30 p.m. on Star Plus, and from 3.30-4.30 p.m. I am generally on the phone with my mother, sister or friends."

- 38 years old, overweight woman

"I prefer sleeping for about half an hour"

- 44 years old normal weight woman

-

"I read books and listen to music during my free time"

- 40 years old obese woman

"My husband gets 2-3 DVD's and we watch movies on our home theater every Sunday and order food from outside."

- 31 years old slightly overweight working woman

"I take my children for their tennis class during my leisure time between 4-5 p.m. 3 days in a week and on the other days I with my children learn vocal music at home."

- 34 years old normal weight woman

Although the leisure activities for most of the women were sedentary in nature, however there was a difference in the way an overweight woman was spending her leisure time as compared to a normal weight woman. Most overweight women preferred watching television and talking on phone whereas, normal women were either taking a short nap or spending time with their children.

(vii) Difficulties in losing weight

Lack of time for physical activity, lack of dietary restraint, lack of company, growing age, joint family, husband, children, in appropriate neighborhood built environment, identification with larger body size were seen as barriers to successful weight loss.

"I have such a hectic job that I do not have time and energy for any kind of physical activity. I will prefer sleeping than walking for that extra 15 minutes"

- 35 years old overweight woman

"I am my own enemy because I cannot say no to food"

- 37 years old overweight woman

"Gradually with age my stamina is reducing. I do not have the strength to go out for a walk. I feel weak and lazy which was not the case earlier"

- 45 years old overweight woman

"Joint Family में रह कर आप आपनी मर्ज़ी से कुछ नही खा सकते। *I have to compulsorily eat what is cooked for all"*

- 35 years old overweight woman

"I have no body to go out with"

- 42 years old woman

"When elders are in the house, relatives keep dropping in and sweets and namkeen have to be served and invariably I also eat"

- 40 years old overweight woman

"When my children were small I used to play with them, they enjoyed my running with them but now time has changed they are teenagers who do not want to be accompanied so my regular outdoor routine has stopped"

- 43 years old slightly overweight woman

"My household responsibilities have increased many times with growing children their school schedule also their coaching classes and on top of that my in-laws keep ill most of the time that I do not have time to go out"

- 37 years old overweight woman

"In South Extension, there is no proper place for walking. Even if I want to walk, I have no place to go except the busy roads, which is not at all safe"

- 36 years old overweight woman

"पहले मैं अपने घर के बाहर ही walk कर लिया करती थी, आजकल हमारे घर के आसपास इतनी construction हो रही है की बाहर walk करना नामुमकिन है।"

- 41 years old normal weight women

"मेरे तो पति मुझे पतला होने ही नही देते क्यूकी वो खुद भी काफ़ी heavy है, और कहते है की हम दोनो ऐसी ही अच्छे लगते है। अगर मैं पतली हो जाती हूँ तो हम दोनो एक साथ अच्छे नही लगेगे ।"

- 38 years old overweight woman

"My in-laws, husband and children make fun of me when they watch me exercising and worrying about my weight. They tell me that I don't have to walk the ramp and will still have to do the household work in which looks is not a criteria. This completely de-motivates me, and I stop doing whatever exercise routine I have started"

- 39 years old overweight woman

"All my friends and colleagues are heavy so we all do not feel the need to reduce weight because everyone believes in enjoying and eating rather than spending time on exercise"

- 39 years old woman

Thus for most of the women the motivating factors and barriers for weight reduction and maintenance were similar. It was seen that family friends and built environment acted as enhancers for some and the very same family, friends and built environment were posing as deterrents in the task of weight reduction for other women. The difference between the two set of women, i.e. maintainers and gainers was the ability to overcome the obstacles coming in the way of the weight reduction.

The salient findings of Focus Group Discussion are as under

1. Most women were concerned about their overweight status.

2. Most of the women were concerned for cosmetic reasons but some women were also concerned about their general well being and health.

3. Overweight status was largely explained by reasons such as genetics, post-partum weight gain, habit of nibbling calorie dense snacks while watching television or talking on telephone, eating little leftovers from child's plate in order to avoid wastage of food, frequent partying, overweight husband, sedentary lifestyle, stress at home and work place. But, some overweight women could not any reason behind their weight status because they were not only eating less but also leading an active life.

4. Most of the women with desirable body weight were able to keep excess weight at bay because most of them had worked out a right combination of physical activity and regulated eating in their life. Also, like over weight women, factors like genetic and stress were responsible for normo weight in case of some women.

5. Most overweight women were successful in losing weight but failed to maintain reduced weight.

6. Family was a motivating factor for maintaining normal weight status, but was also quoted as a barrier in weight reduction by overweight women.

7. Active participation in play with children helped in maintaining weight was felt by all women. But women in middle age or whose children had grown old felt that the nature of activities with older children were more sedentary and required less active participation.

8. All women felt that appropriate neighborhood built environment was essential for indulging in physical activity and thus weight maintenance.

9. Some form of physical activity like yoga, pranayam, brisk walking etc is effective in maintaining weight even if practiced daily even for fifteen minutes as quoted by most of the normal weight women.

Structured weight loss programs help in immediate weight loss, but are not beneficial if and when discontinued. This was the general feeling of all those women who had tried losing weight by joining a gymnasium or a weight management clinic.

(viii) Conclusion

The focus group discussions regarding body weight revealed that most of the women are conscious about their body weight irrespective of their weight status. However, women who had been able to maintain weight described persistent efforts to ensure adequate physical activity and conscious food consumption. They had been able to resist cultural and family norms regarding food quantity and type. These women had been able to strike a balance between time for themselves and their multiple responsibilities. Also, the "feel good" effect after exercise was felt to be a great motivating factor. Social support was found to be the added key to the success of any weight loss or maintenance program. The built environment contributed to the women who had been able to maintain weight. Moreover women with healthy weight had specific plans like drinking water, eat out less, judicious eating in social gatherings, exercise, etc. On the other hand overweight women cited reasons like lack of time for physical activity or healthy food preparation, inability to resist temptation for eating favourite food, lack of social support, psychological emotional stress and inappropriate built environment for weight gain.

The FGD revealed that a wide variety of factors affect women's weight status such as – family preferences, cultural food patterns, work schedules, social relations, stress and access to food. All women believed that diet and exercise are important for healthy weight but social circumstances act as deterrents in adopting healthy lifestyles.

The clear difference between healthy weight maintainers and overweight women was that the overweight women were lazy, lacked motivation or will-power, and failure to manage time and probably find an excuse. Only onset of a disease ultimately makes them to take remedial steps.

Hence efforts need to be directed towards providing education and understanding on a larger social platform since family preference and support is key to the adoption and maintenance of healthy weight.

Although it was not asked but most of the women felt that such interactions and discussions are good learning experiences rather than structured weight loss program. Therefore, during social gatherings discussions related to methods which work best in maintaining normal weight status should be encouraged.

The broad spectrum of reasons given by the women for excess body weight are in agreement with the known reasons of weight gain by urban women largely leading a sedentary lifestyle. Similar reasons were put forth by Emirati women in the age group of 20 to 60 years in a qualitative study exploring weight management behavior and perception of women who are at increased risk of type-2 diabetes by Ali et al (2010).

5. DISCUSSION

The key objective of the present study was to understand how dietary and lifestyle factors affect the weight status of well to do women (25-45 years) because these factors have a varied effect on varied individuals. The factors have been evaluated and tabulated in Chapter 4 of the study. In this chapter the factors affecting the weight status have been discussed with respect to the four BMI categories i.e. normal (N), pre-overweight (PO), overweight (OW) and obese (Ob).

5.1 EFFECT OF SOCIO-DEMOGRAPHIC FACTORS ON BMI

The socio-demographic profile of the subjects included information on age, education, occupation, religion, type of family and marital status. It was observed that increasing age, higher education, joint family and number of parity were the significant factors affecting the weight status of the subjects.

The mean age of women in N (34.6 yrs) was significantly lower ($p<0.001$) than that of women in PO (37.2 yrs), OW (37.0 yrs) and Ob (37.4 yrs) as shown in table 4.1.1(b). Thus women in N category were younger to those in other three categories. The effect of age on weight has been widely reported by various researchers. In a study by Jain and Singh (2003) on women (n=100; 25-50 yrs) working in sedentary jobs in Jaipur City, reported that women in the age range of 45-50 yrs had the highest percentage (26.3%) of obesity, followed by 15.09% in 35-45yrs and 14.2% in 25-35 yrs.

Wasuja and Siddhu (2002) in their study on age related alterations in energy cost, energy requirement and energy status of affluent women (30-88 yrs) reported significant positive association between weight and age ($r=+0.85$; $p<0.001$) in affluent women of Delhi till 60 years of age, which is in agreement of the observation made in this study that weight increases with age for women (25-45 yrs).

Similar findings were reported by Agrawal and Mishra (2004) in their study on overweight and obese women of North India for covarieates of overweight and obesity, that there is four fold increase (2.9 to 11.8) in obese women from age group of 20-29 yrs to 40-49 yrs. Also, they reported that women in the age group of 40-49 years were two and a half times more overweight than women in 22-29 yrs.

In a study by Stbye et al (2011) on body mass trajectory through adulthood on 9681 adults in Singapore in the age group of 19-49 yrs, reported that body weight of women increases during early and middle adulthood.

Sternfeld et al (2004) examined the relation of aging, menopausal status and physical activity to weight and waist circumference in 3,064 racially/ethnically diverse women in the age group of 42-52 yrs reported that the mean weight increased by 2.1 ± 4.8 Kg for women in mid-life.

Thus, the findings of this study reiterate that women tend to gain weight with age.

In India women's education is linked to her socio-economic status which in turn is linked to her weight status as can be seen in the present study. NFHS-3 (2005-2006) also made a similar observation regarding the weight status, socio-economic status and education.

Agrawal and Mishra (2004) reported a positive correlation between women's education and levels of overweight and obesity in the states of Delhi and Punjab. They reported that levels of obesity increased from 5% to 15% with increase in the level of education from graduation to professional in the state of Punjab.

African American women had higher BMIs at moderate and highest level of education as compared to whites who had high BMI at lowest level of education in a study on bi-racial sample of women at mid-life for race, education and weight change (Lewis et al, 2005).

However, Robinson et al (2004) in their study on impact of educational attainment on the quality of young women's diet reported that lower educational level led to faulty eating amoung the women in UK, which in turn led to weight gain.

In the present study significant number of Ob (29.9%) were post graduates and significantly higher women in OW (57.6%) were professional (table 4.1.2), indicating that higher educational level led to higher BMI. This can be attributed to a fat that better education gives better jobs, which are more sedentary and thus affect the weight status.

In the present study, significantly higher (p=0.002) number of women in OW and Ob category were living in a joint family set up (table 4.1.5). This finding can be explained by the fact that in joint families the chances of elaborate meals and socialising is more, which contributes to increased intake. This explanation gets strengthened by the findings of the focus group discussion (qualitative data), where the overweight women quoted that living with in-laws/in joint family leads to greater socializing and to inability to cook in one's own way.

Similar observation was reported by Ackerson et al (2008) in their study on 76,681 Indian women living in 26 Indian States. It was reported that individual factors like high socio-economic status, availability of labour saving devices and household help has lowered household physical activity, but increased social interactions, which has led to weight gain for women living in affluent urban households.

5.2 HEALTH PROFILE AND BMI

In the present study information about the health profile of the study population was collected with the help of questionnaire cum interview schedule. The health profile of the subjects included information on family history of chronic diseases, weight status of parents, reproductive health, morbidity, self perceived weight status of women in four BMI categories.

Role of Family History

Family history was a significant factor ($p=0.001$) affecting the weight status of women as shown in table 4.2.1. The results in table 4.2.1 revealed that significantly greater number of women in OW and Ob reported family history of chronic degenerative diseases like obesity ($p=0.001$), hypertension ($p=0.001$), heart disease ($p=0.018$) and diabetes ($p=0.041$). Family history of obesity, hypertension and heart disease was also identified as one of the final determining factor ($p<0.001$; OR = 6.43) during multivariate analysis. Thus, pointing towards the significant role of genetic predisposition in the spreading of non-communicable diseases in the community. Van der Sande Marianne et al (2001) in their study on the population of Gambia, concluded that the family history of hypertension, obesity, diabetes and stroke was a significant risk factor for obesity and hyperlipidemia. Likewise in an epidemiological study in Chennai by Mohan et al (2003), it was reported that prevalence of diabetes was higher amongst the subjects who had a positive family history of diabetes. According to Rahilly and Farooqi (2006), obesity tends to co-occur within individuals of the same family. In the prevalence study of obesity, in North Iran, 35.3% of the study subjects had a family history of parental obesity (Tilaki and Hiedari, 2007).

Parental weight status

Parental weight status of the study subjects was a significant factor ($p<0.001$) affecting the weight status of women in the study. Although, this factor is covered under family history, but it needs to be mentioned separately because during the binary logistics multivariate analysis (table 4.12.3), weight status of father came out as a determining factor for desirable body weight of women in the study. It was observed that chance of occurrence of obesity in woman is 3.4 time higher incase her father is overweight. Similar observation was made by Cooper et al (2010) in their study on associations between parental and off-spring adiposity. It was reported that there was a strong parent – off spring BMI association (0.06; 95.0% CI : 0.05), which was unaffected when adjusted for a wide range of lifestyle factors. It was also reported that if parental BMI was 1 unit higher, offspring BMI at 44 - 45 years would be higher by 0.21 and 0.29 units. Other researchers have also reported a positive association between parental and offspring adiposity, which persists into adulthood (Kivimaki et al, 2007; Katmarzyk et al, 2008).

Reproductive Health Variables

Reproductive health variables included information on age of menarche, regularity of menstrual cycle, age of marriage, age at first parity, miscarriage and breast feeding.

The mean age of onset of menarche was lower in women in the three overweight categories, i.e. 12.7 years, 13.0 years and 13.4 years in PO, OW and Ob categories respectively versus 13.5 years ($p<0.001$) in N category (Table 4.2.3.1). Similar findings were reported by Lakshman et al (2008) in their study on age at menarche and risk of diabetes in adults, that age of onset of menarche was significantly lower in overweight women with diabetes than in normal BMI non-diabetic women (12.8 years versus 13.0 years; $p=0.008$). Similarly, a longitudinal growth study performed in Finland that at the age of 31 yrs, the prevalence of obesity in females who reached menarche before the age of 11 yrs was 15% compared to those who reached menarche after 15 yrs of age (Laitinen et al, 2001).

Early menarche has been associated with increased risk of obesity in adulthood because girls with early sexual maturation have longer period of positive energy balance, since sexual maturity is linked to fat accumulation in childhood (Garn,1986).

Regularity in menstrual cycle was reported by all 90 subjects in N. On the other hand, significantly lesser ($p=0.022$) number of women in the three overweight category reported having regular menstrual cycle (Table 4.2.3.2). Similar observation was made by a study on 726 Australian women in the age group of 26 – 36 years that 26% of women in the obese category had irregular menstrual cycles compared with 14% of those with the BMI range of 20-24.9 (Wei et al, 2009).

Age of marriage was also a significant factor ($p=0.001$) affecting weight status. The mean age of marriage of Ob category (23.8 years) was significantly lower ($p=0.001$) than that of N (24.7 years). A cross-sectional and longitudinal association between

BMI and marriage, spouse similarity in BMI was reported due to shared environment (Jeffery and Rick, 2002). Also, in a study on influence of educational level and marital status on dietary intake, obesity and other cardio-vascular risk factors in Hong Kong Chinese population reported lower BMI in both men and women (Woo et al, 1999) who were staying single. For the present study, the women belonging to Ob category got married at a younger age and were possibly less concerned about their weight status after marriage. Also, they had early parity (Table 4.2.3.4), which contributed to their weight gain.

Parity has always played an important role in affecting women's weight status. In the present study, the post partum weight gain was significantly higher (p=0.001) for women belonging to Ob and OW category as compared to women belonging to N and PO category (11.76 kg versus 4.81 kg). Even age at first parity and number of children came out as significant factors for positive weight status (Table 4.2.3.5). Professor King (2000) in her review of physiology of pregnancy, explained that energy in excess of foetal needs has a high potential to be stored as maternal fat because of the overall anabolic milieu of pregnancy. Post partum weight gain as observed from tables 4.2.3.9 (a) and (b) was significantly higher (p<0.001) for OW and Ob women. When the dietary intake pattern of 387 women in the present study during pregnancy and lactation was analysed from the questionnaire, it was found that among the women (19.1%; n=74), who reported consuming fat during pregnancy, none belonged to N (table 4.3.1.1.). Thus, indicating that women in the three overweight BMI categories, i.e PO, OW and Ob, consumed more energy dense foods than their counterparts in N category during the period of pregnancy, which might have led to high post pregnancy weight retention.

Also, Ob women had early parity and number of parity was also significantly higher (p<0.001) for these women (Table 4.2.3.5). This finding was supported by a study of parity-overweight relationship with level of household wealth and the national human development, it was reported that in wealthy women number of parity was positively related to overweight regardless of the level of national human development (Kim et al, 2007). Also, various research studies in the past have pointed to cumulative cycles of post partum weight retention as the mechanism by which parity leads to overweight (Harris et al, 1997; Gunderson and Abrams, 1999; Winkvist et al, 2003; Olson et al, 2003).

Miscarriage is an adverse pregnancy outcome. In the present study more number of women belonging to OW and Ob (40.2%; n=47 and 30.8%; n=36) categories had experienced miscarriage as compared to women belonging to N and PO category (16.02%; n=19 and 12.8%; n=15). Agrawal and Mishra (2004) in their study on North Indian women for the effect of overweight and obesity on adverse pregnancy outcome reported that more overweight and obese women in the age group of 15-29 years have experienced miscarriage and abortion due to still birth (OR=1.57; 95% CI:1.06, 2.33 for overweight and OR=2.10, 95% CI: 1.02, 4.29 for obesity) than women with normal BMI.

Consumption of oral contraceptives as a family planning measure was adopted by significantly higher (p=0.004) number of women belonging to OW and Ob category (55.6%; n=45 and 17.3%; n=14) as compared to PO and N category (17.3%; n=14 and 14.8%; n=12). But duration of intake was not significantly different (p=0.567) for the four BMI categories (Table 4.2.3.7). Weight gain as a side effect of consumption of oral contraceptives was reported by significantly higher (p=0.001) number of women belonging to OW and Ob category. Although, review of literature does not support this finding because in a study on evaluation of impact of an oral contraceptive on body weight concluded that intake of oral contraceptive has a negligible effect on body weight status (Endrikat et al, 2001).

Co-morbidites

Association of obesity with poor health is well documented. Obesity has a more pronounced effect on morbidity than on mortality, it increases the probability of the individual suffering from obesity related morbidity and disability (Astrup, 2005; AHA, 2008).

The secondary data obtained from the women, reinforced the above fact. All the diagnosed cases of pre-hypertension, hypertension, impaired fasting blood glucose and high cholesterol belonged to either OW or Ob BMI category, but none to N and PO BMI category. However, significant number of women in PO and N category had blood cholesterol level in the at-risk range of high cholesterol i.e total cholesterol between 170-199 mg/dl (Table 4.2.5). This can be explained from the dietary fat intake data (Table 4.9.1), in which it was seen that the mean fat intake of the women belonging to N and PO category was much higher than the desirable limit of 40 g/d, and was comparable to the mean fat intake of women in OW and Ob. Also, significantly higher percentage of women in N was ovo-vegetarians and was consuming egg daily (Table 4.4.1 and 4.4.2).

In a similar study by Agarwal (2005) on role of lifestyle and diet in emerging obesity among Indian women and its impact on their health status, reported that 48% of obese and 32% of overweight women reported poor health status as compared to 25% of women with normal BMI. Specific morbidities like asthma, high cholesterol and thyroid problem was reported by 10% of obese women, 4-5% overweight women and just 1% women with normal BMI. Also, in the same study, it was observed that there was not much change in the health status over the years amongst the women with normal BMI.

Self perceived weight status

Erroneous perception of bodyweight can have important health and behavioural implications. Therefore in the present study women in the four BMI categories were inquired about their own perception of their body weight status. It was revealed that majority of the women (86.6%; n=335) correctly perceived their weight status. Thus indicating that women are realistic and sensitive to their body weight status, which is an important factor in any weight management programme. In a similar study by Serdula et al 1999, on prevalence of attempting weight loss reported that higher percentage of overweight females (43.6%) were attempting weight loss as compared to males (28.8%).

Paeratakul et al (2002) compared the self perception of overweight in the study population according to sex ,race/ ethnicity and socio- economic status and also compared the self perception of overweight among individuals classified as normal weight, overweight and obese. Multiple logistic regression showed that the odds ratio of perceived overweight was significantly higher in women, whites and individuals with higher body mass index, higher income and higher education. Self perceived weight status was also identified as a determining factor affecting desirable body weight of women in the study (Table 4.12.3) during the binary regression analysis. Thus, indicating that correct perception of weight status helps in maintaining normal body weight. In the present study, significantly higher ($p < 0.001$) number of women belonging to OW(58.6% ; n = 119) and Ob (22.7% ; n = 46) category were trying to lose weight by various methods as compared to women in N (9.4% ; n = 19) and Po (9.4% ; n = 19) category (Table 4.2.9). Thus, indicating that more number of overweight and obese women were dissatisfied with their present weight status. In a study across European Union regarding body image perception and satisfaction with current image revealed that the subjects who were most content with their body weight were females who were underweight (Mc Elhone et al,1999).

5.3 EFFECT OF DEITARY PATTERN ON BMI

Our genotype plays a substantial role in the development of obesity but it alone cannot be implicated for the current obesity epidemic. Behavioural and environmental factors are equally important (Racette et al, 2003). Intake related behaviours that have been linked to obesity include frequent consumption of meals at fast food and other eating establishments, consumption of large portions at home and at restaurants, consumption of energy dense foods, such as high fat, low fibre foods, and intake of sweetened beverages. These behaviours occur in an environment in which energy dense food is abundant, relatively inexpensive, easy to obtain and easy to eat with minimal preparation (AHA, 2008). Therefore, in the present study the food behaviour of the 387 women in the four BMI categories was studied with respect to past dietary behaviour as well as present dietary behaviour, which included information on food preference, type of diet, frequency of eating out, snacking and other food habits.

5.3.1 Food Behaviour

Food behaviour of the women in the four BMI categories can be discussed with the help of three terms i.e restraint, dis-inhibition and hunger, as suggested by Stunkard and Messick (1985).

Dietary restraint is defined as a tendency to consciously restrict food intake either to prevent weight gain or to promote weight loss by control over both energy intake and types of foods eaten (Pirke and Laessle, 1993).

Dis-inhibition is the tendency to overeat in presence of palatable foods or other dis-inhibiting stimuli such as emotional distress (Lowe and Maycock, 1988).

Hunger is the susceptibility to perceived body symptoms that signals the need for food (Lowe and Maycock, 1988).

Dis-inhibition was significantly higher ($p<0.001$) for women belonging to OW (47.6%; n=146), Ob (25.1%; n=77) and PO (17.3%; n=53) categories as compared to women belonging to N (10.0%; n=31) in terms of overeating (Table 4.4.7). Similar to this observation, Hays et al (2002) reported a strong association between dis-inhibition and BMI ($r=0.27$; $p<0.001$) in their study on eating behaviour correlates of adult weight gain and obesity in healthy women aged 55-65 years.

Snacking behaviour is another dis-inhibiting behaviour, which was observed to be significantly higher ($p<0.001$) for women in OW (47.9%) and Ob (22.3%) as compared to just 16.0% in N (Table 4.4.16.1 and 4.4.16.2). Forslund et al (2005) in their study on snacking frequency in relation to energy intake and food choices in obese men and women compared to a reference population reported that obese group snacks more frequently compared to the reference group ($p<0.001$) and women more frequently than men ($p<0.001$). It was not only the frequency, but also the type of snack consumed by women in OW and Ob that influenced their weight status. Consumption of energy dense snacks like potato chips, namkeens, samosa and pakora was significantly higher ($p<0.001$) for OW and Ob (Table 4.4.141 and 4.4.14.2). Piernas and Popkin (2010) in their study on snacking prevalence in U.S adults between 1977 and 2006 reported that prevalence of snacking increased significantly from 71% to 97%. Also, the contribution of snacks to total energy intake increased from 18% to 24% ($p<0.001$). The study reported that commonly consumed food sources were found to be salty snacks, candies and sweetened beverages.

Dietary restraint in the study population was evaluated with the help of fasting pattern as well as regularity of taking the three main meals by the women in the four BMI categories. It was observed that significantly higher ($p<0.001$) number of women belonging to OW (42.2%; n=92) and Ob (29.8%; n=65) were observing fast as compared to N (22.5%; n=49) and PO (5.5%; n=12) BMI category (Table 4.4.9.1). Also, significantly higher ($p=0.001$) women in OW, Ob and PO were skipping one or more of their three main meals (Table 4.4.4) as compared to almost none in N. It is a well known practice to reduce food intake in order to lose weight, but it is normally accompanied by reduced physical activity, which prevents weight loss.

In a recent study on rhesus female monkeys for change in energy balance during dieting revealed that there was a significant decrease in the daily activity level with no significant weight loss (18 ± 5.6% decrease, $p=0.02$). It was concluded that a diet induced decrease in physical activity is the primary mechanism that the body uses to defend against diet induced weight loss (Sullivan and Cameron, 2010).

Therefore, dietary restraint in the form of fasting/dieting or skipping meals does not lead to weight loss. In the study on eating behaviour and weight gain by Hays et al, 2002 suggested that dietary restraint may be a critical moderator for adult weight gain.

The third most important aspect of food behaviour is the susceptibility or response to hunger. This aspect was studied in terms of eating speed, tendency to overeat at meal times, and eating in between meals. Significantly higher ($p<0.001$) women in OW and Ob were fast eaters than women in N (Table 4.4.5). Also, significantly higher ($p=0.001$) women in OW and Ob were overeating at meal times for a wide variety of reasons, but the most significant reason for overeating was hunger. The multivariate analysis revealed that overeating by women when hungry was also a determining factor for desirable body weight of women in the study. It was observed that significantly higher ($p<0.001$) women in OW and Ob were eating in between meals as compared to N (Table 4.4.6). These results clearly point towards the fact that possibly overweight and obese women in the study were unable to regulate their eating. On one hand, they were showing greater dietary restraint by fasting and skipping meals, but on the other hand, they overate on being hungry and also ate in between meals. Conversely, women in N reported having a fixed appetite at all times (Table 4.4.6).

Therefore, we can say that the overweight/obese status of the study subjects was due to faulty food behaviour like overeating, skipping main meals, snacking on energy dense food products and eating in between meals. On the other hand, the women in N category had more effective food behaviour in terms of dis-inhibition, restraint and hunger. They were more regular with respect to taking of the three main meals along with regulated appetite.

5.3.2 Diet Composition

Positive energy balance is explained by a simple fact that when energy intake is more than energy expenditure. But, energy in the diet is provided by three macronutrients viz carbohydrates, fats and proteins. In the body most storage fat comes directly from dietary triglycerides, but excess dietary carbohydrates and proteins are also converted to fatty acids in the liver by lipogenesis (Gee et al, 2008). Therefore, diet composition in terms of the three macronutrient, eating out pattern, intake of convenience foods, which are normally energy dense along with the frequency of consumption of soft drinks, intake of sugar in a cup of tea or coffee and monthly consumption of fats and oils was mapped for the women in the study.

In the present study it was observed that the mean energy intake of women belonging to OW category (1998 Kcal/d) was significantly higher ($p<0.001$) than the mean intake of women belonging to N (1634 Kcal/d). Similarly, the mean fat intake for OW category (67.5 g/d) was significantly higher ($p<0.001$) as compared to that of N (58.1 g/d) category. However, it was also observed that the mean energy (1690 Kcal) and fat (58.1 g/d) intake of women belonging to Ob category was comparable to N category (Table 4.9.1). Surprisingly, the mean energy and fat intake of women belonging to PO category (1876 kcal/d; 64.8g/d) was significantly higher ($P<0.001$) than both N and Ob category (Table 4.9.1). Even the mean carbohydrate intake of OW (289.5 g/d) and PO (260.9g/d) was significantly higher ($p<0.001$) than that of N (229.5 g/d) and Ob (229.8g/d) category. The analysis of the dietary intake among study sample clearly indicates that women in the OW and PO categories are over consuming than women in the N category. However, no significant difference in the dietary intake of N and Ob category can be explained by underreporting by Ob, change in dietary behaviour whereby significant number of Ob women were restricting intake of fried foods and sugar (Table 4.4.10 and 4.4.12), skipping meals, nibbling and snacking behaviour. Yao et al (2003) in their study on relative influence of diet on body composition in urban Chinese adults reported that dietary fat was not significantly associated with BMI but other factors like dietary variety, frequency of restaurant food consumption were significantly ($p=0.001$) associated with body fatness.

The data on eating out (Table 4.5.1) and consumption of convenience foods (Table 4.4.15.1 and 4.4.15.3) clearly point towards the fact that significantly higher ($p<0.001$) OW and Ob women were eating out and were also using convenience foods more frequently (Table 4.4.15.2). It is a well known fact that convenience foods are normally prepared with hydrogenated trans fats or saturated fats to improve their shelf life. Also, foods prepared in restaurants are made with the motive of greater palatability, which normally comes from greater use of fats and oils along with spices. Thus greater use of convenience foods and higher frequency of eating out by the women in the OW and Ob category had a significant influence on their weight status. In the Nurses Health Study on the association of dietary fat and weight gain among adult women ,it was reported that although there was a weak positive association between total fat intake ($\beta=0.11$) and weight gain but there was a strong positive association between weight gain and increased intake of trans fat, animal fat and saturated fat . Also women who were overweight at baseline were more susceptible to weight gain with greater dietary fat consumption, however, there was no meaningful relationship between percentage of Calories from fat and weight gain among non-overweight women (Field et al, 2007). Restaurant meals are considered to be high in energy density than home prepared meals. Consequently regular consumption of high energy dense diets can lead to passive over consumption and increase in body weight (Rastrolla et al, 2008). In a study by Mc Cory et al (2000) on dietary determinants of energy intake and weight regulation in healthy adults reported that positive association between the frequency of consuming restaurant foods and body fatness ($r=0.36$, controlled for age and sex). It was reasoned out that restaurant food is high in fat and low in fibre thus energy intake is promoted by high ratio of energy intake to food weight. Also restaurants serve a variety of palatable foods in large portions.

The consumption of soft drinks like carbonated drinks, fruit juices etc was significantly higher ($p<0.001$) for OW and Ob categories as compared to N (Table 4.4.17 a & b). Duffey et al (2010) reported that consumption of sugary drinks is associated with higher risk of high waist circumference ($r=1.09$; $p<0.001$) in a study on relation between consumption of Caloric beverages and cardio metabolic risk factors. Sugar sweetened soft drinks and fruit juices have been identified as one of the dietary contributors to overweight and obesity (WHO, 2003). This report stated that each can of soft drinks consumed per day increases the risk of being obese by 60%.

It is a general practice that during fasting or dieting, women tend to increase their fluid intake, which is normally in the form of beverages. As observed in the present study that the consumption of soft drinks like carbonated drinks by Ob and OW were significantly higher as compared to that of N (Table 4.4.17 b). Also, the intake of sugar in a cup of tea or coffee was significantly higher for OW women (Table 4.4.16) as compared to other three categories at the rate of 2 tea spoons per cup. The data clearly indicates greater consumption of sugar in the form of beverages by OW and Ob women, which explains their present weight status.

The fat consumption data in terms of monthly consumption of fat and frequency of consumption of fried foods among women in the four categories revealed that the mean intake of refined oil, desi ghee and butter was significantly higher ($p<0.001$) for OW and Ob as compared to N (Table 4.4.18). Also, significantly higher ($p<0.001$) women in OW (33.7%) and Ob (37.6%) were consuming fried foods atleast once a week as compared to just 9.9% in N (Table 4.4.19). Various research studies in the past have reported that dietary fat and sugar can promote obesity without excessive energy intake because they carry more energy in even small amounts (Herberg et al, 1974; Oscai et al, 1984, 1987; Levin et al, 1986; Miller et al, 1990; Mc Cory et al, 2000; Rastrolla et al, 2008; and Merchant et al, 2009).

Thus, the consumption pattern of women belonging to OW and Ob category in terms of eating out consumption of convenience foods, sugar and fat was more indulgent than that of N. The findings of quantitative dietary patterns were corroborated by the qualitative data collected by FGD in which the overweight and obese women particularly stated that they cannot control the sight of their favourite, which was most often sugar or fat based like chips, bhujiya, kurkure. People normally tend to over eat high fat foods not only because they taste good but also even small amount of food packs so many calories. In comparison non over weight or normal weight women had found various ways of avoiding energy dense foods even when surrounded by them. Like a normal weight woman told during an FGD that since she has to socialize a lot but she takes care that she does not eat too many snacks and drink too many cold drinks. So, she takes a glass of carbonated drink which she keeps sipping till the end and same about her snacks plate. In this way she avoids eating energy dense snacks and people around never get to know because her plate is always full and her glass is never empty. (Section 4.12- FGD).

Role of dietary carbohydrate and protein

Apart from the quality and quantity of the fat consumed, the kind of carbohydrate and protein sources are also important factors influencing weight status. In the present study both qualitative and quantitative data revealed that consumption of refined carbohydrate was higher amongst women belonging to OW and Ob category. The quantitative data obtained from the 24 hour dietary recall revealed that although there is no significant difference between the mean carbohydrate intake of N and Ob category (Table 4.9), but the in depth analysis of the consumption pattern of type of snacks (Table 4.4.14.2), food preferences while eating out (Table 4.5.2.1) and type of convenience foods consumed (Table 4.15.3) by the women in the 4 BMI categories revealed that the consumption of snacks like potato chips, namkeen, convenience foods like pasta, noodles and preference for fast foods while eating out was significantly higher ($p<0.001$) for OW and Ob as compared to N. Qualitative data from FGD revealed that most obese and overweight women were eating refined carbohydrates because their children want to eat such food items and they do not feel like cooking separately for themselves. Even when eating out, the overweight and obese women reported that they ate what their children preferred. In contrast most of the women in the N category preferred selecting a less energy dense items and even guided their children to choose a healthy option like having a vegetable topping pizza rather than a plain cheese pizza.

Merchant et al (2009) in their study on carbohydrate intake and overweight and obesity among healthy adults concluded that consuming a low carbohydrate (< 47% energy) diet is associated with greater likelihood of being overweight or obese among healthy free living adults. Participants who ate more fruits and vegetables were less obese whether or not their diet were high fat or low fat compared with participants who ate fewer fruits and vegetables. Overall diet quality, together with physical activity is related to weight maintenance. Energy dense food are rich in refined carbohydrates and unhealthy fats. Snack food items and soft drinks make up the majority of energy dense foods, while energy density is low in fruits and vegetables poultry, fish and whole grain (Ledikwe et al, 2006; Drewnowski, 2007). Although obesity is recognised as a disorder of energy balance, but the debate on controlling obesity hangs on achieving optimal balance of macronutrients. AHA (2008) dietary guidelines advocate a daily intake of macronutrients with carbohydrates ≥ 55% of dietary energy, fats limited to ≤ 30% of dietary energy and protein ≤15% of energy. In the present study carbohydrates accounted for 56.1% of dietary energy for N, 55.5% for PO, 57.9% for OW and 55.1%for Ob BMI category, which was significantly different ($p<0.026$). The contribution of protein energy was significantly higher ($p<0.001$) for N category (13.8%) as compared to PO (12.3%), OW (11.6%) and Ob (12.8%) category (Table 4.9.1). Thus, pointing towards the role of dietary protein in weight regulation. The review of literature gave the following reasons for supporting the role of proteins in the regulation of food intake and healthy body weights.

Protein suppress food intake more than fats or CHO and do so more than which can be accounted by their energy content alone (Barkeling et al, 1990; Porrini et al, 1997; Latner and Schwartz, 1999; Anderson and Moore, 2004; Wardlaw and Hampl, 2007).

Protein make a stronger contribution to satiety and delay the return of hunger compared with fat and CHO (Hill and Blundell, 1986; Rolls et al, 1988; Marmonier et al, 2000; Flint et al, 2000; Laymane et al, 2003; Woodend and Anderson, 2003; Stubbs et al, 1999).

High protein diets support the maintenance of lean body mass under circumstances of energy restriction, thereby promoting weight loss primarily as adipose tissue (Hong and Layman, 1984; Gautsch et al, 1998; Anthony et al, 1999; Layman et al, 2003).

Protein digestion leads to the stimulation of many physiological and metabolic responses known to be involved in food intake regulation (Layman et al, 2003; Anderson and Moore, 2004; Layman, 2004)

The evidence regarding the role of protein in weight regulation is important but equally important is the choice of protein in the diet. Normally all good sources of proteins are animal based which are low in fibre and high in saturated fat, which is linked to increased risk of CVD (Mc Carty, 2000). Thus, it is important to balance the source of dietary protein from both animal and plant sources. The source of protein in the diet can be judged from the type of diet consumed by the individuals. In the present study an insight in to the dietary preference for vegetarian and non-vegetarian diets revealed that significantly higher (p=0.001) number of women belonging to OW (43.7%; n=59) and Ob (35.6%; n=48) category were non- vegetarians as compared to N (8.1%; n=11) category (Table 4.4.1).

However, significantly higher (p= 0.001) number of women belonging to N (45.6%; n= 57) category were ovo-vegetarians as compared to women in PO (18.4%; n=23), OW (36.0%; n= 45) and Ob (none) category (Table 4.4.1).

Since egg is an excellent source of protein but not calcium therefore, it can be said that the high protein intake of N category was due to the consumption of egg. The frequency of consumption of egg and flesh food amongst the women in four BMI categories revealed that significantly higher (p=0.001) number of women belonging to N category were consuming egg / flesh food daily or at every alternate day as compared to women in other three categories. Thus pointing towards the fact that high protein intake helps in weight regulation.

Since there was no net difference in the energy and fat intake of N and Ob group, the reason of imbalance in weight can be possibly due to faulty dietary practices.

Similar observation was reported by Kushner and Choe (2010) in their study on prevalence of unhealthy lifestyle patterns among overweight and obese adults. They concluded that unhealthy lifestyle patterns in diet and exercise are highly prevalent in overweight and obese populations.

The data from FGD (Chapter 4.12) revealed that women were aware of correct dietary practices but barriers like unhealthy food choices of family members especially children and poor self control created the difference between normal weight and overweight. Unlike the olden days, today's women whether working or staying at home prefers speed scratch cooking i.e. combining fresh ingredients with processed food or eating out. The consumption pattern has shifted from traditional Indian meals to fast foods which are rich in trans fat, saturated fat, refined Carbohydrates, sodium and sweeteners. Traditional Indian beverages like *Jal Zeera, Nimbu Pani, mango panna* etc have been replaced by calorie dense beverages like carbonated drinks and packed juices. In the present study the dietary practices of women belonging to N category were significantly different from that of OW and Ob categories but it was the women in PO category who it seems are following the path of weight gain due to faulty dietary practices. Therefore dietary counselling for women belonging to PO category regarding the role of diet needs to be initiated.

Also, in a Quebec family study on risk factors for adult overweight and obesity, Chaput et al (2009) found that in adults (aged 18-64 years), short sleep duration, high dis-inhibition eating behaviour, low dietary calcium intake, high susceptibility to hunger behaviour, non-participation in high intensity physical exercise, high dietary restraint behaviour, non consumption of multi-vitamin and dietary supplements, high dietary lipid intake, and high alcohol intake were all significantly associated with overweight and obesity in the cross-sectional sample (n=537).

5.4 ANTHROPOMETRIC AND BODY COMPOSITION FACTORS AND BMI

On ANOVA, the mean body weight of N was significantly lower (p<0.001) than PO, OW and Ob (Table 4.7.1). Similar findings were reported by Nande et al (2010) in their study on influence of obesity on body measurements and composition in adult women belonging to minority community. They observed a difference of 10.97 kg, 25.97 kg and 30.03 kg between normal versus overweight, normal versus obese grade–I and normal versus obese grade-II respectively. In the present study the difference in mean body weight of N versus PO, N versus OW and N versus Ob was 5.7 kg, 12.14 kg and 26.61 kg respectively. These figures are a cause of concern because having a BMI in the overweight or obese range is associated with an increased risk of developing hypertension, high-cholesterol, type-2 diabetes and coronary artery disease (Kopelman, 2007). Also, Kozak et al (2011) reported that overweight and obesity in early adulthood is adversely associated with self reported physical health related quality of life (HRQOL) twenty years later but was not associated with mental health. Thus, reflecting that the body weight needs to be managed for not only healthy adulthood but also a disease free old age.

In the present study, the prevalence of general obesity (BMI $\geq$ 30) was 20.67%, whereas, the prevalence of overweight was 40.31% (table 4.7). Gopinath et al (1994) reported obesity prevalence of 33.4% in adult urban female population of Delhi. Asthana et al (1998) reported obesity prevalence of 30.24% among the women of Varanasi City of Uttar Pradesh. Wasuja and Siddhu (2002) reported overweight and obesity prevalence rate of 60% among well to do urban women of Delhi in the age group of 30-49 years. Zargar et al (2000) reported obesity prevalence of 23.69% in Kashmiri women. On the other hand Bhadra et al (2005) reported obesity prevalence of 17.45% in Bengali women of Kolkata City in West Bengal. In the global context, it was observed that the prevalence percent of 20.67% in the present study was broadly in agreement with the prevalence of more affluent countries of the West like Canada (25.6%) (Johnston et al, 2004), Germany (27.0%) (WHO, 2000[1]) and USA (24.8%) (WHO, 2000[1]). However the present study was not designed for prevalene.

The obesity rate of present study when compared with that of affluent Asian countries like Japan (2.6%) (WHO, 2000[1]), South Korea (3.2%) (WHO, 2000[1]) and China (0.86%) (WHO, 2000[1]) was much higher.

In the recent study by Balarajan and Villamor (2009) on trends in the prevalence of overweight – obesity and underweight among women of reproductive age in three South Asian countries of Bangladesh, Nepal and India between 1996 and 2000, observed that the prevalence of overweight and obesity increased from 10.6% to 14.8% in India. Thus according to this prevalence rate and all India prevalence of 15.0% (NFHS-3, 2005-2006), the prevalence of obesity reported in the present study is much higher, but was lower than the overall prevalence of 34% in women of Delhi according to NFHS-3. However, these are prevanance rates which cannot be compared wwith the sample as the sampling with primarily purposive. Obesity rate of 20.67% in the present study was also lower than the prevalence rate of 47.4% in Indian women as reported by Deepa et al (2009) in their study on prevalence and significance of generalized and central body obesity in an urban Asian Indian population of Chennai.

BMI and Body Fat Percent

WHO (2000[1]) defines obesity as a condition of abnormal or excessive fat accumulation in adipose tissue, to the extent that health and well being may be impaired. The mean body weight of the women in the four BMI categories clearly points towards the presence of excess body fat in the three overweight categories i.e PO, OW and Ob. Also, the review of literature supports the fact that there is a gradual accumulation of body fat during adulthood, but the extent of accumulation differs widely (Speakman and Westerterp, 2010; Mc lean, 2005; Apovian, 2010; Heber, 2010; Ito et al, 2001; Kyle et al, 2001; Kyle et al, 2006).

In the present study using the PBF value $\geq$ 30.0% and $\geq$ 35.0% for classifying overweight and obesity, respectively in women (Dudeja et al, 2001; Siddhu, 2004) revealed that 67.2% (n=260) women were obese, of which 14.6% (n=38) belonged to PO, 54.6% (n=142) to OW and 30.8% (n=80) to Ob BMI category, but none belong to N category (Table 4.8.2.1). Bhadra et al (2005) reported obesity prevalence of 36.53% on the basis of PBF (cutoff $\geq$ 30.0%) in a study of obesity among adult Bengalee Hindu women. Using the PBF cutoff of $\geq$ 30.0% for classifying overweight women, it was observed that 66.3% of N were overweight (Table 4.8.2). Thus, reflecting that the body fat is in excess not only in women belonging to OW, PO and Ob BMI categories, but also in women belonging to N category. In the present study, there was a significant difference ($p<0.001$) amongst the four BMI categories with respect to the PBF. The mean PBF of PO, OW and Ob category was respectively 36.1%, 41.3% and 50.1% as compared to 30.5% for N category (Table 4.8.1). Similar observation was made by Nande et al, 2010 in their study on affluent Indian women belonging to minority community. They reported a significant difference ($p<0.01$) between the mean PBF of normal BMI group (27.23%) and that of obese group (37.95%). It was noted that both Bhadra et al study and Nande et al study were done on minority community respectively in East and South of India; therefore, in those studies the PBF value of normal BMI group was lower than that of the present study because in the present study majority of the women were North Indians belonging to Hindu Punjabi community. The difference can be attributed to ethnic and geographical variations.

BMI and Fat Free Mass Index (FFMI) and Fat Mass Index (FMI)

BMI is a sum of FFMI + FM (Schutz et al, 2002). Expressing FFM and FM as percentages of body weight or by weight has limitations, as a person that carries more weight in lean tissue may be incorrectly classified as possessing and undesirable body fat. Also, fat mass (FM) and fat free mass (FFM) have different health effects. When only BMI is used as a criterion of nutritional status, these divergent relationships cannot be distinguished (Hull et al, 2011; Heymsfield et al, 2005; Allison et al, 1997; Van Itallie, 1990). Therefore, FMI and FFMI of the study subjects was calculated from the body composition data.

The mean FMI and FFMI of Ob (16.37 kg/m2; 16.21 kg/m2) category was significantly higher ($p<0.001$) than not only N (6.57 kg/m2; 14.94 kg/m2) category, but also from OW (11.24 kg/m2; 15.89kg/m2) category (Table 4.7.3). Thus, clearly indicating that excess weight of women in Ob category was largely due to excess body fat. When the FMI and FFMI data of this study was compared with that of Caucasian population (Kyle et al, 2003), it was observed that the mean FMI of normal BMI (18.5 – 24.9 kg/m2) Caucasian women was 4.4 kg/m2 as compared to 6.57 kg/m2 for N BMI (18.5 – 22.9 kg/m2) category in the present study. This indicates that for the same BMI Indian women, even with normal BMI range, have higher body fat than the Caucasians. This finding is fully supported by the data of various other researchers that Indians in general have a genetic phenotype characterised by a low BMI and high body fat with upper body adiposity (Kurpad, 2003; Siddhu, 2004; Yajnik 2004; Rush et al, 2009). Similar trend was observed for other categories also i.e. women in the present study belonging to OW and Ob BMI categories had higher mean FMI values at 11.24 kg/m2 and 16.37 kg/m2 respectively, as compared to that of Caucasian women in overweight (10.9 kg/m2) and obese (13.9 kg/m2) BMI category in a study by Kyle et al (2003) on healthy white men and women.

BMI and Abdominal Obesity

It is not just the amount of fat but also its distribution that determines the risk associated with obesity. Abdominal or visceral fat (android obesity) is associated with the cardio-vascular risk factors of the metabolic syndrome (WHO, 2000; Wang, 2003). Abdominal fat mass can vary in any individual for the same BMI and total body fat (Gopalan, 1998). In the present study, abdominal obesity was studied among the women belonging to the four BMI categories with respect to waist circumference (WC), waist hip ratio (WHR) and waist stature ratio (WSR). On the basis of cutoffs for WC ($>$ 80.0 cm), WHR ($>$ 0.8) and WSR ($\geq$ 0.5), the prevalence of abdominal obesity amongst the women in the study population was 56.6% (n=219), 31.0% (n=120) and 66.6% (n=258) respectively.

This indicates that more than half the women in the study were abdominally obese. In the Indian women's health study, the overall prevalence of central obesity among women between 25-64 years of age was 55.0% (Hariram and Talwar, 2005). Similarly, Deepa et al (2009) reported a prevalence of abdominal obesity in Indian women on the basis of WC as 56.2%, which is quite close to the prevalence rate of 56.6% in the present study.

The data on occurrence of abdominal obesity among women in the four BMI categories revealed that significantly higher ($p<0.001$) percentage of women in OW and Ob had abdominal obesity as compared to N (Table 4.7.2.1, 4.7.2.2 and 4.7.2.3)

Similarly, in a study by Gupta et al (2009) on identification of cardio-vascular risk factors in North India reported the prevalence of abdominal obesity as 32.3% in females (n=1042; 15-39 years) on the basis of WHR.

The present study also confirms the rising trend of occurrence of abdominal obesity in urban affluent women. This is a disturbing trend because abdominal obesity has been confirmed to be one of the most important CVD risk factors and the health risk associated with central obesity have been reported to be even more prominent than general obesity as measured by BMI (Seidell et al, 2001; Dobbbelsteyn et al, 2001; Misra and Vikram, 2003; Yusuf et al, 2005; Ko and Tang, 2007; Misra and Khurana, 2009). Also, Goodpaster (2005) reported that greater visceral adipose tissue is independently associated with metabolic syndrome in older men and women, particularly among those of normal body weight.

Misra and Virkam (2004) reviewed the topic of metabolic syndrome and obesity in Asian Indians from the data-bases in pubmed and Current contents and from non-indexed publications of the medical research and governmental institutions in India. They concluded that high prevalence of excess body fat, adverse body fat patterning, hyper-triglyceridemia, and insulin resistance beginning at a young age have been consistently recorded in Asian Indians irrespective of their geographic locations.

5.5 EFFECT OF ENERGY EXPENDITURE, ENERGY STATUS AND PHYSICAL ACTIVITY ON BMI

In human beings energy expenditure is a continuous process irrespective of the conditions encountered which is in steep contrast to the process of food intake, which is carried out in a discontinuous manner. Therefore, it is important to understand the Energy Expenditure (EE) in humans. Energy Expenditure is a total of three components i.e. energy spent on Basal metabolism or (basal metabolic rate, BMR), energy spent on physical activity and energy spent on thermogenesis i.e the response of the body to a variety of stimuli including food, cold, stress and drugs. In the present study energy expenditure of the women in the four BMI categories was studied in terms of BMR and physical activity.

BMR and BMI

BMR cannot be practically measured therefore it has been replaced by Resting metabolic rate (RMR), which is 10% - 20% higher than the BMR (Frary and Johnson, 2008). However, the term BMR has been used for the calculated RMR in the study. The BMR of the women in the four BMI categories was significantly different ($p<0.001$). The mean BMR increased positively with the increase in category i.e the mean BMR of N category (1224 ± 34.9 Kcal/d) was lowest, followed by the mean BMR of PO category (1278 ± 44.3 Kcal/d), then by OW BMI category (1327 ± 56.4 Kcal/d) and finally the highest was of Ob BMI category (1452 ± 73.1 Kcal/d) (Table 4.10.1). This can be explained by the fact that obese (Ob) people have greater amount of fat-free mass (FFM) as well as fat mass (FM) than the people with normal BMI, and since 60% – 85% of RMR can be attributed to FFM (Nielsen et al, 2000), RMR is typically higher in obese (Pi-Sunyer, 1991).

The mean FFM and mean FM of women belonging to Ob 39.4 kg; 39.7 kg) and that of OW category women (38.3 kg; 27.0 kg) was significantly higher than the mean FFM and mean FM of women belonging to N BMI category 36.8 kg; 16.2 kg). Therefore, the BMR of the Ob group was higher by 228 Kcal/d than the BMR of N group. Although, some research suggests a strong genetic component of RMR and implicates low RMR as a predictor of weight gain (Bogardus et al, 1986; Bouchard et al 1989; Ravussin et al, 1988), however other studies have shown no contribution to RMR to future obesity risk (Weinsier et al, 1995; Seidell et al, 1992; Katzmarzyk et al, 2000).

Similar RMR pattern was reported by Johanssen et al (2008) in lean (1505 ± 109 Kcal/d) versus obese (1601 ± 109 Kcal/d) white healthy pre-monopausal women.

Total Energy Expenditure (TEE) and BMI

In the present study the mean TEE (total energy expenditure) of Ob category was significantly higher ($p<0.001$) at 2243 Kcal/d as compared to N (2079 Kcal/d) category (Table 4.10.1). Previous research by Maffeis et al (1993) explained this difference by the fact that the energy cost of conducting weight bearing movements is greater in obese persons than equivalent movements in non-obese persons. Also, Pi-sunyer (1991) reported that obese people expend more Kcal/d than non-obese persons. Therefore the difference in the energy expenditure of N and Ob category is largely due to the difference in the BMR and not due to greater physical activity by the women in the Ob category. In case of the other two overweight categories i.e. PO and OW, the energy expenditure of PO (2000 ± 117.9 Kcal/day) was significantly lower ($p < 0.001$) than N and also that of OW (2069 ± 145.2 Kcal/day) category (Table 4.10.1). The TEE of OW was also lower than that of N but not significantly. This data indicates that women in PO and OW category are expending less energy than women in N category. This fact is further substantiated by the data on mean time spent in daily activities i.e. obligatory, discretionary without exercise, exercise and residual activities. It was observed that the mean time spent in daily activities was significantly lower ($p < 0.001$) for PO (982.3 minutes), OW (987.4 minutes) and Ob (992.6 minutes) as compared to N (1031.2 minutes) category. However the three overweight categories were not significantly different (ANOVA) from each other with respect to the mean time spent in discretionary activity (Table 4.10.4). Butte et al (2003) reported that women in the normal BMI group spent significantly more time doing household and occupational activities ($p=0.02$) than women in low and high BMI group in the age range of 20-40 years. Welle et al (1992) in their study on EE in normal and overweight women reported that the significantly higher values of TEE in overweight women became un-significant when adjusted for body size and composition of both the normal and overweight group. They observed that the higher 24 hour energy expenditure and TEE values observed in the overweight women were attributable to the higher BMR and energy cost of activities. Also, Dugas et al (2011) reported no significant difference in the energy expenditure of adults in developing and industrialized countries.

The energy expenditure data when compared with the energy intake data of these four categories revealed that the energy imbalance of Ob was highest (-562 Kcal) and was least for OW (-71.1 Kcal) (Table 4.10.5 b). Swinburn et al (2009) reported total energy intake as the main driver for higher body weights in modern populations. They reported that heavier people have significantly higher imbalance ($p < 0.0001$).

Physical Activity and BMI

Physical activity refers to any bodily movement produced by skeletal muscles that results in energy expenditure (Timperio et al, 2008). The contribution of physical activity is the most variable component of total energy expenditure (TEE). The energy expended for physical activity is of two types, activity thermogenesis (AT) and Non exercise activity thermogenesis (NEAT). AT is the energy expenditure during sports or fitness exercise whereas, NEAT refers to the energy expended during activities of daily living (Levine and Kotz, 2005). NEAT includes all household, occupational, residual and discretionary activities without exercise. It excludes energy expenditure on sleeping and eating. Rather than AT it is the contribution of NEAT and sedentary lifestyle which promotes obesity (Levine et al, 2006). In the present study, all the subjects were considered sedentary, since none exercised regularly or participated in occupations that required extreme exertion. Also, the energy intake of N (1634 ± 234 Kcal/d) BMI category was not significantly different ($p=0.168$) from that of Ob (1690 ± 378 Kcal/d). Thus the significant difference ($p<0.001$) in their body weight status i.e positive balance can be attributed for difference in the physical activity, particularly the daily routine activities.

Physical activity has four dimensions i.e frequency, intensity, duration and type (Timperio et al, 2008). In the present study, it was observed that the self reported time spent in sitting was significantly different ($p<0.001$) for the four BMI categories. The mean sitting time was highest for OW (8.7 hours), closely followed by Ob (8.4 hours) and PO (7.6 hours) category, whereas the mean sitting time for N category was 5.9 hours (Table 4.6.7.6). When calculated as a percentage of an average day, OW women sat 36.25%, Ob women sat 35.0%, PO women sat 31.66% and N category women sat 24.6% of the time. The mean time spent in standing by women in the four BMI categories was significantly higher for the women belonging to N (6.9 hours; $p<0.001$) BMI category. The mean time spent in walking by women in four BMI categories was highest for women belonging to N (3.6 hours), but it was not significantly different the other three BMI categories. These results point towards the duration aspects of the physical activity. It appears that women belonging to N category are spending enough time in activities which help in maintaining weight as compared to women in the other three BMI categories. The present study found a significant positive association ($r=+0.184$; $p<0.001$) between sitting time and BMI categories.

NEAT behaviour differed significantly between lean and obese individuals, as the obese subjects spent an average of two hour per day more in seated position compared with their lean counterparts (Levine at al, 2005). This study result was quite similar to the results of the present study. Similarly Johannsen et al, 2008 reported that obese women sat 53% (800 minutes) and lean women sat42% (600 minutes) of the time. Also, they observed that obese women stood 11% (200 minutes) and lean women stood 20% (300 minutes) of the time.

The mean PAL value of the women in the four BMI categories gave an idea of the intensity of physical activity indulged in by the subjects. In the present study the mean PAL of N (1.69 ± 0.08) was significantly higher ($p<0.001$) than that of Ob (1.55 ± 0.10), OW (1.56 ± 0.08) and PO (1.57 ± 0.07) (Table 4.10.1). The difference in the mean PAL values of the four BMI categories further supported the discrepancies between the women in the three overweight categories and the women in N category with respect to the energy expended in being active. Various studies have found that the subjects who were active enough to raise their PAL to > 1.7 were better able to maintain their weight than those below that threshold (Weinsier et al, 2002; Adams et al, 2003; Johannsen et al, 2008). Also, FAO/WHO/UNU (2004) has recommended a PAL Value of 1.75 to prevent obesity.

In India, household activity like cooking, dusting, washing etc require considerable energy expenditure, which also constitutes the NEAT behaviour. The data from the present study revealed that not only more number of women belonging to N (44.5%; n=61) category (Table 4.6.3.1 and 4.6.3.2) were performing household activities like cooking, washing clothes and the like, but were also engaged in these activities more frequently (daily) as compared to women belonging to Ob (11.7%; n=16), OW (29.2%; n=40) and PO (14.6%; n=20) category. Also, performance of household activities was observed with respect to the kind of domestic help employed. Presence of full time domestic helpers was linked to non performance of household activities. It was observed that significantly higher ($p<0.001$) number of women belonging to OW (47.6%; n=121), Ob (23.2%; n=50) and PO (16.9%; n=43) BMI category had permanent full time helpers as compared to just 12.2% (n=31) women belonging to N (Table 4.6.2). This also clearly indicates that the women belonging to the three overweight categories were expending less energy in household activities as compared to women belonging to N category.

From the results in the present study, we can conclude that the energy expended in NEAT activity was lower in women belonging to PO, OW and Ob BMI categories as compared to N category.

Similar results were reported by Agrawal, 2005. It was reported that 77% women experienced increase in their BMI status with a full time maid. Also, 48% women gained weight among those not involved in performing household activities like cleaning and washing as compared to 25% who were performing household chores.

In the present study, the sedentary behaviour of the women belonging to the three overweight categories was further highlighted with respect to the time spent in exercise. The results show that the mean time spent in exercise by the women in N category is significantly higher ($p<0.001$) than that of their counterparts in other three overweight categories. While women in N category spent an average of 30.4 ± 26.9 min/d in exercise, the women in OW category (21.1 ± 21.6 min/d) followed by women in PO category (20.5 ± 21.2 min/d) and least time spent by women in Ob category (17.6 ± 21.3 min/d) (Table 4.10.3). Physical activity in terms of exercise is known to have a beneficial effect on health. Field et al, 2010 noticed that females who exercised ≥ 5 days per week and limited portion sizes gained 1.9 kg less that those females who were just dieting or those who were combining low fat diet with exercising at least once a week. AHA scientific statement 2008, reiterated the beneficial effect of regular physical activity. To make lasting changes in weight, adults must engage in 30 – 60 minutes of moderate to vigorous physical activity ≥ 5 days per week.

Similarly, May et al, 2010 suggested an inverse relation between physical activity level and subsequent weight and waist circumference change in both men and women.

Slentz et al, 2004 reported a significant ($p<0.05$) dose – response relationship between amount of exercise and amount of weight loss and fat mass.

In the present study, the women belonging to Ob, OW and PO category were neither actively indulging in household activities nor were exercising, therefore it can be said that these women were spending their leisure time in sedentary activities like watching television or operating computer and the like. The self reported data on mean time spent in watching television revealed that women in Ob (95 minutes), OW category (90 minutes) and PO category (70 minutes) were spending significantly higher ($p<0.001$) time than women in N (55 minutes) category (Table 6.7.7).

According to the two studies of Robinson and Goodbey (2005)[1 & 2], watching television during free time normally displaces exercise or physically active leisure pursuits because adults have only a few hours daily for discretionary activities.

Time spent in watching television has been associated with deleterious effects on physical activity, diet and BMI (Meyer et al, 2008; Tsintsifa et al, 2006).

On the other hand Otten et al (2009) reported that reduced television viewing produced a statistically significant ($p=0.02$) increase in energy expenditure after three weeks of intervention.

In the present study, the time spent in television viewing was positively and significantly ($r = +0.284$; $p<0.001$) associated with BMI. Also, the multivariate logistic regression analysis identified time spent in television viewing (Table 4.12.3) as one of the determining factors affecting desirable body weight of the women in the study. Thus, it can be concluded that in the present study, watching television might have substituted for time spent in more physically active activities like outdoor play with children. In this study, results showed that although women in the four BMI categories were not significantly different with respect to playing outdoor games with children, however there was a significant difference ($p<0.001$) with respect to the mean time spent in outdoor play. Exercise time was inversely and significantly correlated ($r = -0.197$; $p<0.001$) with BMI. The percentage of women playing outdoor games in four BMI categories was respectively OW (39.3%; n=44), N (30.4%; n=34), Ob (20.5%; n=23), PO (9.8; n=11) (Table 4.6.7.5.1). However, the mean time spent in playing outdoor games by women in four BMI categories was highest for N (4.4 hrs) followed by OW (3.4 hrs), Ob (3.3 hrs) and least for PO (2.5 hrs) (Table 4.6.7.5.2).

Therefore, it can be said that sedentary behaviour of television viewing in the three overweight categories was largely contributing to their present weight status. This study result also takes support from the fact that women in the three overweight category reported greater snacking behaviour than women in N BMI category. This study result clearly implies that snacking behaviour is promoted by television viewing which leads to reduced physical activity and weight gain. Similar to this result, Meyer et al (2008) associated high television exposure with 20% to 30% greater odds of being above the median for serving of salty snacks, sweets and sweetened drinks and below the median for fruit and vegetable servings in U.S adults. Television exposure was also cross–sectionally associated with a greater odds for being overweight or obese. Also Tsintsifa et al (2006) observed lower fat consumption in men and women spending more time in activities comparable to walking at a leisurely pace and light household work ($r = -0.264$: $p < 0.01$).

Sleep also plays a fundamental role in health maintenance. Epidemiologic study suggests that chronic sleep deprivation pre disposes to mortality, heart disease, diabetes and obesity.

Sleep was positively but not significantly ($r = +0.092$; $p=0.071$) correlated in the study. Since the present study was not specifically designed to study sleep duration; therefore, the information on habitual sleep duration was obtained by a question on bedtime / wake time. On the basis of this information sleep duration was calculated for women in four BMI categories. It was observed that the average sleeping time for the study sample was 7.4 hours (443.5 ± 82.1 min). The mean sleeping time of PO, OW and Ob category was 7.7 hrs, 7.55 hrs and 7.45 hrs respectively; whereas, that of N BMI category was 6.9 hrs. (Table 4.6.7.7). On the basis of this data we can say that increase in sleep duration leads to weight gain. Landerdale et al (2009) classified sleep into short duration (<6 hrs), average duration (6-7.5 hrs) and long duration (>7.5 hrs). They reported that short duration sleepers gained 0.73 kg more than those reported sleep > 7 hours. This positive association between short sleep duration and BMI was observed only in the cross-sectional analysis. The study observed no longitudinal association between sleep measurement and change in BMI.

Patel and Hu (2008) reviewed research articles related to sleep duration and increased weight. According to them, five studies reported no association between short sleep duration and increased weight. While six studies found evidence that long sleep durations are associated with increased weight resulting in U-shaped curve between sleep duration and weight. Also, one study reported reduction in weight due to short sleep duration.

The women in the present study were falling between short and long duration sleepers. However, the women in the three overweight categories are sleeping more than the women in the N category. Thus, the sleeping trend in the present study points towards a U-shaped relationship between sleep and BMI. Similar to this result, Chaput et al (2007) reported greater weight gain in both short sleepers (5-6 hrs) and long sleepers (9-10 hrs) in their study on adult aged 21-64 years from families oversampled for obesity in Canada.

On the basis of the physical activity and energy expenditure data we can say that the women belonging to N category (table 4.10.2), although sedentary with minimal planned physical activity were able to maintain normal weight. So it appears that they are engaging in amounts of activity recommended for avoidance of weight gain i.e. 30-60 minutes of moderate intensity activity per pay with a PAL of $\geq$ 1.7 (Johannsen et al, 2008). Also, the data suggests that the difference between the N and Ob category is due to the difference in daily activities of low intensity rather than high intensity. Weinsier et al (2002) suggested that low intensity physical activities like walking, using the stairs and gardening might not be sufficient for inducing weight loss, but they can support weight maintenance. On the other hand sedentary behaviour like erratic sleeping, viewing television and sitting has adverse effect on the BMI.

5.6 DETERMINING FACTORS FOR DESIRABLE BODY WEIGHT STATUS OF WOMEN (25-45 YRS)

Out of the host of factors found significant for body weight status (Table 4.11.1), it were the six factors which came out as the final determinants of body weight status of women in the study (Table 4.11.3). When these factors were studied along with the observations of the focus group discussion (Chapter 4.12), it clearly emerged that out of the six determining factors, three factors which related to the behaviour, like the tendency to overeat when hungry, loner sitting time and longer time spent in television viewing. These factors were also quoted as causative of weight gain by participants of the focus group discussion like an overweight participant stated that she never overeats, but while watching television or talking on the telephone, she finishes of the packet of biscuit or namkeen in her hand. Also, other participants felt that while talking and working on computer, they invariably lose count of the amount of food eaten. Thus, in general it was observed that most overweight/obese women had poor self control with respect to eating snacks while watching television and in social gatherings and were more sedentary. They had habit of giving exeucses of overeating and not exercising.

The other three determining factors i.e overweight status of father, family history of obesity, hypertensions, heart disease and self perceived normal weight status also highlighted the need for a behavioural change. This change was observed in the dietary and lifestyle behaviour of N (n=90), and normal weight participants of FGD.

Women with normal weight status were able to maintain their weight status because –

1. They were conscious about the amount and type of food eaten by them.

2. They consciously restricted themselves as well as their children from watching excessive television. They also avoided keeping snacks handy with them while watching television or while working on computer.

3. They preferred not to overeat under any circumstance. They followed fixed meal and portion size. They do not overeat when hungry.

4. They rarely allowed their children to decide what has to be eaten instead they guide/influence their children towards a healthy choice which suits their palate as well as their body while eating out and at home.

5. They were doing some basic yoga exercises like pranayam for just 15 min daily.

6. By purposely making a small change in their daily routine i.e sleeping a little early at night and getting up earlier in morning to enable them to devote time in morning exercise.

7. They had found ways to avoid overeating and do exercise within their social enviornment.

8. A trend of gaining 3-4 Kg of post partum weight was observed for women in N category in comparison to a post partum weight gain of 7-10 Kg in OW and Ob category (table 4.2.3.8). Thus it can be said that a port partum weight gain of 3-4 Kg will keep a woman in normal weight category, and any gain beyond this would make her overweight.

9. A per annum weight gain of 2-3 Kg is easier to lose/gain as observed for women in N. But, gain of 7-10 Kg per annum is difficult to shed and makes to woman overweight (table 4.2.8).

10. For normal weight women sitting time is less and do more household/occupational course, which require standing and walking.

11. Normal weight women consumed more furits and vegetables, were ovo-vegetarian and had lower fat especially ghee even during pregnancy and lactation.

12. Even being sensitive or becoming conscious of one's normal weight helps in maintaining weight because this sensitivity brings with it the desired behavioural change, which is responsible for the difference between women with desirable body weight and excess weight.

In the study it was observed that a wide variety of factors affect women's weight status such as – family preferences, cultural food patterns, work schedules, social relations, stress and access to food. All women believed that diet and exercise are important for healthy weight but social circumstances act as deterrents in adopting healthy lifestyles.The clear difference between healthy weight maintainers and overweight women was that the overweight women were lazy, lacked motivation or will-power, and failure to manage time and probably find an excuse. Only onset of a disease ultimately makes them to take remedial steps.

Thus, the study helped in identifying dietary, behavioural and lifestyle factors important for maintaining desirable body weight among urban affluent women by both qualitative and quantitative approaches. The six significantly determining factors from quantitative study were in agreement from qualitative factors especially long sitting time, television viewing time and tendency to overeat as factors contributing to weight gain. The self perceived normal weight status (OR-57.03) brought significant behavioural changes, which were evident in FGD narrations also. It is quite possible that tracking one's own self image flags the sequel of behaviour changes which ensure normo weight status.

CPSIA information can be obtained
at www.ICGtesting.com
Printed in the USA
LVHW082359051222
734629LV00016B/1142

9 781805 459828